NURSING AND SPIRITUAL CARE

NURSING AND SPIRITUAL CARE

Edited by

Olly McGilloway BA, SRN, BTAcert, DN(Lon), RNT
Director of Nursing Studies
New University of Coleraine
Coleraine, Northern Ireland

and

Freda Myco PhD, BA, SRN, BTAcert, RNT
Associate Professor of Nursing
University of Lethbridge
Alberta, Canada

Harper & Row, Publishers
London

Cambridge
Hagerstown
Philadelphia
New York

San Francisco
Mexico City
São Paulo
Sydney

First published 1985
Harper & Row Publishers Ltd
28 Tavistock Street
London WC2E 7PN

British Library Cataloguing in Publication Data

Nursing and spiritual care.
　　1. Care of the sick——Religious aspects
　　I. McGilloway, Olly　　II. Myco, Freda
291.1'78321　　RT42

ISBN 0-06-318310-2

Typeset by Activity Limited, Salisbury, Wilts.
Printed and bound by Butler & Tanner Limited,
Frome and London.

This book is dedicated to Connie, Anne and Mary

This book is dedicated to Connie, Anne, and Mary.

CONTENTS

LIST OF CONTRIBUTORS

Aparna Bhaduri, Professor, RN, RM, MSc, EdD
Department of Nursing Research, Rajkumari Amrit Kaur College
of Nursing, New Delhi, India

Patrick Darcy, SRN, RMN, DN(Lon), RNT, Cert Ed
Director of Nurse Education, College of Mental Health Nursing,
Purdysburn Hospital, Belfast, Northern Ireland

Liam Donnelly, Father, BA, CC
St Finlough's Church, Ballykelly, Northern Ireland

Alison Kitson, BSc(Hons), SRN, DPhil
Lecturer in Nursing Studies, University of Ulster, Coleraine,
Northern Ireland

Rosemary McCavery, BSc(Hons), SRN, ICUcert
Formerly Staff Nurse (ICU), Craigavon Hospital, Northern Ireland

Charles McDaid, SRN, RMN, RMND, BTAcert
Nursing Officer, Stradreagh Hospital for the Mentally Handicapped, Londonderry, Northern Ireland

Olly McGilloway, BA, SRN, BTAcert, DN(Lon), RNT
Director of Nursing Studies, University of Ulster, Coleraine,
Northern Ireland

Freda Myco, PhD, BA, SRN, BTAcert, RNT
Associate Professor of Nursing, University of Lethbridge, Lethbridge, Alberta, Canada

Julia Neuberger, Rabbi, MA
South London Liberal Synagogue, Prentis Road, Streatham,
London

Abdullahi Wando, RN, DipAns, Cert Adv Nurs Adm
Nursing Officer, II, Ministry of Health General Hospital, Minna,
Niger State, Nigeria.

PROLOGUE

Modern medical research addresses itself to the mechanisms of life and death, and health and illness, rather than to the meaning of their occurrence. Such research tends not to accept that the sacred might be located in any of the spheres it investigates. Fox (1976) claimed that medical research tries to detach itself from what it regards as the biasing effects which the ideas of specific religious traditions might impose on investigation.

The influence of medicine has invaded areas previously dominated by religion and, at times, seems to have almost relegated the spiritual aspects of health care to nothingness. This effect will be seen to vary across clinical settings. Yet there can be no doubt that, in the main, spiritual care has featured with decreasing frequency alongside advances in medical science and specialization. As the health system becomes more scientific and differentiated the care of the individual becomes more impersonal and segmented (Field 1971).

Modern medical thought is resolutely anti-magical in intent, if not always in fact (Bellah 1964). Consequently, medicine today is akin to that of State religion yesterday, in that it has an officially approved monopoly of the right to define health and illness and to treat disease (Friedson 1970). The institutions and theories of medicine define the standards of health and abnormality which shape what people feel and think about themselves and, when necessary, use State power to legitimize and extend such authority.

Despite existing in the age of space technology and microchips, health concepts and practices for the most of society contain cultural traditions which have evolved from antiquity. If one accepts that culture is a particular form that survival, coping, and viability take in a given human group, then, as Horobin (1978) claimed, health has always been an essential part of human culture and cannot be logically separated from it.

How people come to identify health problems, why they are concerned about them and their consequences, are influenced by their social context, as well as by the character of the medical care system. The willingness of the patient to cooperate, and his response to treatment, will be affected by the extent to which the medical context conforms or clashes with socio-cultural expectations. In many respects, modern medicine is itself a derivative of modern socio-economic development. Galdston (1981) claimed that the ways in which the physician serves the patient, in whatever setting, and in what order of relationship, both contractual and economic, are determined not by the medical profession, but by the socio-economic forces dominant at a given time. He claims that, 'the socio-economic system prevailing now, has obtained such complexity that patterns of medical practice are not entirely suitable, or entirely effective'.

While scientific excellence may be considered an appropriate criterion for testing reliability, personal and social attributes cannot be overlooked; attributes such as nationality, class, political persuasion and religion cannot be ignored. The ultimate aim of the social way of life is the fullest possible development of all the capacities of the individuals who make up society; thereby giving the fullest possible satisfaction in the form of the complete personality. This demands that both the doctor and the nurse recognize that each human being has intrinsic worth or value, which may be neither ignored nor discounted in the patient's care, irrespective of his achievements.

Respect for a person implies a positive concern for his welfare independent of the kind of person he might be. This demands an active sympathy from the nurse, coupled with a sense of moral obligation. Obligation implies the antithesis of inclination (Harris 1968). It does not necessarily follow that inclination and obligation cannot coincide, rather obligation to act is a form of constraint to be adopted irrespective of inclination. Moral obligation, therefore, can be said to be obligation in the absence of any likely threat or punishment if action is not taken. According to Harris (1968), the source of moral obligation appears to be value, and its object the realization of value — that is, the greater good. Nursing activity has its origins in moral obligation. For the nurse to get close to the patient, she has to be able to tolerate and come to terms with things which often produce fear, conflict, and sometimes disgust in the patient and in others. In such situations, both nurse and patient may seek comfort in religion. While most patients have some form of religion, it is often not enough to relieve their anxiety; to support them through phases of denial, isolation, anger or depression, which are frequent responses to illness. Very few individuals respond as a total stereotype of their religious, or indeed cultural group (Sampson 1982). Early in their careers, nurses may experience incongruity between formal religious practices and the need for spiritual comfort among patients. The religious obligations demanded by the different world faiths can be learned from textbooks alongside other theoretical knowledge. But the reassurance, understanding, or experience which some patients seek demands an individual and human approach from the nurse, which cannot be obtained from any textbook; only from within herself, and from her identity as a human being. A nurse who cannot understand, or sense any spiritual worth in herself will not be able to value spiritual worth in the patient in her charge.

The aim of this book is to heighten awareness of spiritual comfort as a major component in patient assessment, and to help in the promotion of the caring aspects of the nurse's role in health care provision. It does not seek to proselytize any one religion, nor to repudiate any individual belief that the reader may hold — it seeks to promote rather than to destroy. It attempts to challenge the reader to explore his or her own attitudes and beliefs about religion, as well as the need for, and implementation of, spiritual care in illness. In doing so it has been necessary to try to place the subject in a wider perspective than has, arguably, been attempted before. However, to cover all possible contributions to spiritual care would be unrealistic within the purview of one book. The reader may find himself or herself in agreement with some parts of the text, and disagreeing, perhaps even vehemently, with other parts; it is doubtful that all will be read placidly and with serenity. If, however, the reader proceeds to examine ways in which spiritual needs are assessed and catered for in any one particular environment with which they are familiar, then the objectives of the authors will have been achieved. No apology is made for any repetition among contributors; each chapter is singular and individual and if certain themes recur, from authors with different backgrounds and from different parts of the world, this surely emphasizes the importance of those particular concepts for spiritual well-being in health or illness.

The chapters are loosely grouped into a framework of three sections. The first of these focuses on philosophical issues, following a broad overview of Man's spiritual needs, in association with medicine, over the centuries. Chapter 2 describes the main religions and their basic concepts and philosophies. Chapter 3 attempts to provide the perspective of the non-believer to such issues as life and death, while the concept of suffering through illness is explored in Chapter 4. The role of alternative care, as practised in the art of faith healing, is brought into focus in Chapter 5.

The second section of the book deals with the ritualistic side of religion and concentrates on the four most common religions, namely Christianity, Judaism, Hinduism and Islam. Each of the contributors to this section is a member of the faith concerned and is involved, directly or otherwise, in the illness situation.

The third section of the book is written by nurses with specialist knowledge of the individual areas of care, namely acute, long-term, mental health, and mental handicap care. Chapter 10 uses the intensive care unit as a focus for discussion of spiritual needs in acute illness, and this is followed by a contribution into the needs of the chronically sick and the elderly. The close relationship between religion and mental health is discussed in Chapter 12 while the importance of recognizing the spiritual needs of the mentally handicapped closes this section of the book.

The subjective nature of religion and spiritual need must be appreciated, but this is not sufficient reason for nurses and other health workers to continue to underestimate the importance of religion and spiritual care to the well-being of the patient and his or her family.

References

Bellah, R N (1964) Religious evolution, American Sociological Review, 29: 359

Field, M G (1971) The health care system of industrialised society: the disappearance of the general practitioner and some implications, in E Mendlesohn, J I Swazey and I Taviss (Editors) Human aspects of biological innovation, Harvard University Press

Fox, R C (1976) The sociology of modern medical research, in C Leslie (Editor) Asian medical systems: a comparative study, University of California Press

Friedson, E (1970) The profession of medicine: a study of the sociology of applied knowledge, Dodd, Mead

Galdston, I (1981) Social and historical foundations of modern medicine, Brunner, Mazel

Harris, E L (1968) Respect for persons, in R T De George (Editor) Ethics and society; original essays on contemporary moral problems, Macmillan

Horobin, D (1978) Medical hubris, Churchill Livingstone

Sampson, C (1982) The neglected ethic: cultural and religious factors in the care of patients, McGraw-Hill

PART ONE

THE PHILOSOPHY OF
RELIGIOUS EXPERIENCE AND SPIRITUAL CARE

CHAPTER 1

RELIGION, MAGIC AND MEDICINE AS A RESPONSE TO SPIRITUAL NEED: AN HISTORICAL OVERVIEW

Origins of religious symbols

The hospital ward is hushed. A student nurse pushes a patient in a wheelchair toward the day room, where other patients have already assembled. The ward sister is arranging flowers and candlesticks on either side of a wooden cross. The minister of religion dons his regalia, lights the candles and offers each patient a text bearing a religious portrait. He prepares to begin a Christian communion service.

Such an event represents a familiar scene in many hospital wards and usually invokes a sense of well-being both in staff and in patients. Implicit in this sense of well-being is a feeling of continuity, of hope for the future, in an environment frequently oppressed with doubt and insecurity. Few present at such a service, however, are likely to dwell on the individual symbols of the ceremony; the origins of the elements which have evolved from antiquity, and which have been bound to the social well-being and health of mankind since the dawn of history. Painting, fire, wood, wine and regalia are among the symbols reflecting the spiritual needs of Man long before the Christian era. A few words about such symbols might serve to bridge the centuries.

The origins of cave paintings are obscure. Scientists have some notion who painted them, but little idea as to why. Whether early man decorated his habitat for pleasure, or if such painting had spiritual meaning is not known. Theories have been put forward that drawings of wild animals were intended to placate the spirit of the hunted, or to fascinate them into captivity. However, none of the rock paintings yet discovered depicts a medical scene. Other forms of drawings, or statues, have been discovered in prehistoric temples across Europe, many of which appear to relate more directly with human life factors such as fertility. The use of holy paintings, relics or statues remains a prominent feature of many of the modern religious practices.

Fire, wood and other elements were ritualized into village ceremonies from the time Man began to form stable communities based on agriculture rather than hunting. Such ceremonies involved seeking protection from misfortune, both for animals and for humans. Kemp (1935) relates that in Slavonic villages, each Spring, cattle and villagers would be made to cross streams, or walk between two ceremonial bonfires, or even go through a tunnel of earth and tree roots constructed to imbibe properties of purification. Wood was frequently worshipped in the form of sacred trees, in sacred groves, with offerings tied to branches to supplicate favour from the Spirit based in the tree. The Christian ceremony of baptism, Moslem ritual washing before prayer, and the lighting of candles are examples of elements with ancient connotations having been incorporated into modern religious ceremonies.

Nurses and patients often wear Christian crosses, Star of David or St Christopher pendants around their necks or pinned to clothing. Amulets, or talismans, were in common use in ancient and medieval societies, and their use in communities separated for centuries by geographic barriers indicates ancient and strong human belief in such symbols. Basically, all talismans can be divided into two types: one prophylactic or strengthening, and the other worn to repulse evil forces. Most were hidden among the owner's clothing to strengthen their power.. Tattoos also had their origin in protective symbolism, as well as decoration.

Food and drink have always held an importance beyond their physiological benefits. The use of alcohol had a place in many ancient cults, from Osiris to Dionysus, and was eventually adopted into the Christian church as part of the communion service (Sigerist 1962). To ancient man the transformation of dead vegetable matter, and parts of animals into living substance, appeared as a mystery, and the act of eating assumed ritual as well as nutritional significance. Acts of cannibalism were performed to assimilate the warrior spirit of the vanquished into the victor. Food, and food offerings, still retain important religious significance. Harvest festivals, fasts such as Ramadan, and communion bread hold both thanksgiving and penitential meanings. Food is usually blessed by saying of prayers, or grace, prior to eating.

Although the Bible attributes the custom of dressing to original sin, dress and decoration has adopted status and symbolic meaning in various religions. Clerical collars, saffron robes and nuns' habits serve to distinguish the religious from the secular. Sumptuous decoration or specific pieces of attire, e.g. a bishop's mitre, have been used for centuries to establish hierarchies within religious groups.

A final example of the incorporation of ancient symbols into modern religious practice is the wayside cross or shrine. These originated in the art of cairn building. When a wrongdoer could not be found, it was common practice in European villages to throw stones in a pile at the roadside, outside the village, as a curse on the wrongdoer. The more stones placed on the cairn, the greater the curse. Cairn building in high places has always been popular among travellers; possibly to ward off evil. Roadside cairns were eventually replaced by crosses, shrines and holy wells, but few hikers today can resist adding a stone to each cairn they pass on a lonely moor — for luck?

Ancient civilizations

The primitive concept of misfortune, in health and disease, was primarily magical. It contained elements of religion but in early civilizations, before records began, it is difficult to draw the line between magic and religion (Sigerist 1962).

Primitive man was surrounded by a hostile environment, every manifestation of which he tended to invest with mysterious forces. To live in harmony with such a world, he resorted to magic as a means of obtaining power over his surroundings. Sickness meant disharmony, that a stronger power had taken command, and health could return only when that power, or spirit, had been placated or banished. The primitive medicine man, or shaman, was much more than just physician/priest to his community. He was also the historian of the tribe, frequently its leader in war, and sometimes even the rain-maker. His functions tended to be sporadic and incidental. He was not usually someone inflicted with psychotic illness, rather he would have had to be very much in touch with the realities of his time. Nor could he have survived long had he been a quack or charlatan.

Rather he must have been of above-average intelligence, possessed knowledge of remedies that cured common ailments and have been a good psychotherapist.

Physical therapies such as baths, hot mud, massages, herbs and poultices were taken or applied as part of magic rituals. Incantations accompanied these activities to increase the supposed power of the remedy, and probably the belief of the patient in it. The use of modern medical terminology, with its origins in Latin or Greek, can be used to impress today's patient as to the superior knowledge of the physician whose skill he seeks.

Modern civilization is said to have its origins in the Middle East with the development of farming techniques. Here the accent shifted from magic to religion. Only when Man had reached this stage of development did the circumstances of his existence allow the cumulative growth of a transmissible medical culture (Galdston 1981). Babylonian culture was an elaborate system of religious medicine (Sigerist 1962). It adopted the belief that all disease came from the Gods, and the task of the priest/physician was to discover and interpret the intention of the deities so as to placate them. However, the role of healer was still open to anyone who wanted to help the sick. In ancient Babylon, the sick were often carried to the market place, where they solicited counsel from anyone who knew anything about their complaint. Gradually, such 'centres', where those seeking help met those offering help, developed into sacred temples. The first Babylonian physicians were priests. They dealt with internal illnesses, especially mental affliction, which was attributed to demonic possession, and treated by magicoreligious methods. Later, in the Babylonian era, lay physicians were introduced. They attended patients suffering external pathology, including trauma, which they treated with natural remedies. The conduct of the lay physician was dictated by the Code, or Law of Hammurabi, which was written about 2100 BC.

The Babylonians believed that the stars were divine and possessed superior intelligence and, consequently, that everything in the Universe had a purpose (Alexander and Selesnick 1966). The menstrual cycle in women and the exacerbation and remission of certain diseases were thought to be governed by the cyclic activity of celestial bodies. Some drugs were used, and incantations were prominent. However, throughout history, few incantations were ever written down, much as the prayers of patients are not part of a modern medical textbook. Nevertheless, to the patient they are as important as his medical treatment.

In ancient Egypt the practice of medicine became more restricted and professionalized, but still dominated by priests. Early medical treatises, though few in number, illustrate the growing interdependence of religion and medicine in this era. Both the Edwin Smyth papyrus, (*circa* 1600 BC), which deals mainly with surgical matters, and the Ebers papyrus (*circa* 1500 BC), which concentrates on internal disease, include mixtures of magical incantation, prayers and practical action. The Egyptians were influenced both by Oriental and by African cultures. Where Oriental influence dominated, mysticism and priestly medicine held sway; while contact with African civilizations prompted a more empirical approach.

Imhotep, the first recorded Egyptian physician (*circa* 2850 BC), became deified as a god of medicine. At Memphis, a temple was built in his name, which became both a hospital and a teaching centre, where incubation or dream healing was practised — pre-dating similar practices among the Aesculapian cult in Greece. While attending the temple, patients were encouraged to occupy their time with recreational activities; an early form of occupational therapy.

Egyptian physicians had little anatomical knowledge. They believed that the body was governed by specific spirits, which corresponded with those found in the environment. For example, the bones and flesh of the body corresponded with the soil, the heart was related to the sun and to fire, and the breath was equivalent to the wind.

Greek civilization

Religion and magic are seldom mentioned in Greek medical treatises and, when they occur, they are usually discussed in a negative sense (Temkin and Temkin 1967). From the fifth century BC, Nature came to be seen as the dynamic power; independent of any divine manifestation. An individual disease was thought to have a nature of its own, but such a nature did not have to contradict the gods because it was created by them and, therefore, could be seen as divine in itself. The existence of divine power in Nature meant that the world was not governed by chance alone, but by intelligent and recognizable laws. This concept of causation stimulated early scientific enquiry. The Greeks sought to explain their world through the doctrine of teleology. They believed that all natural processes were determined by an end to which they were directed. They sought to explain the Universe in the light of final purpose. Consequently, physicians, such as Hippocrates, refused to try to intervene in what seemed hopeless or terminal cases.

The search for equilibrium with Nature led to the Greek fascination with physical fitness. As Osler (1948) pointed out, 'In the golden age of Greece, medicine had a triple relationship, with science, with gymnastics, and with theology'. The Christian belief separated God from Nature, and Nature was no longer seen as an animate form. Thus effects that were seen by the Greeks as natural and empirical came to be looked upon with suspicion and, consequently, ignored by the 'modern' physician.

The Greek physician believed in the power of prayer but did not rely on prayer alone. He did not advise it, but he never sought to prevent the patient seeking divine help — especially when he was seriously ill. However, it was considered to be offensive rather than reverant in Greek society to ask help of the gods. The pious man was expected to express openly only his gratitude. This belief led to the adoption of incubation or dream healing. The sick person was brought to the temple and he was cured, or the way to his cure was revealed to him in his dreams by the gods. Different gods became associated with different conditions. For example, in Sparta, those suffering eye conditions hoped for the help of Athena Ophthalamitis. Priests were the only interpreter of 'divine' dreams, for which they relied on experience rather than argument. Physicians were excluded from dream interpretation, and they did not have the authority to object to the miracle cures claimed to have been performed by the gods.

Many such temples, which eventually stretched from Britain to the Middle East, were dedicated to the deified physician Aesculapius. Perhaps the most famous of these centres was at Epidaurus, in Greece, where a whole complex of buildings was erected around the shrine. Baths, hostels, theatres and restaurants met both spiritual and secular needs of patients and their attendants. A hot bath followed by a vigorous massage helped to promote bodily relaxation before sleep, while attending a comic or tragic play at the theatre could allow an outlet for the emotions.

The physical and spiritual progress of the patient through the temple can be likened to the three phases which anthropologists identify with any ritual concerned with the rites of passage. These three phases are: separation, margin (or *'limen'*, Latin for 'threshold') and aggregation. In the first phase, by entering the temple, the patient becomes separated from the norms of conventional society. Entering the second, or liminal phase, freed from all institutional relationships, he feels a sense of fellowship with all mankind; a sacred or holy state. The final phase of reintegration involves adopting, once again, a clearly defined system of rights and obligations in his society.

Patients who felt their condition was improved, or cured, by this experience showed gratitude by leaving behind a replica, or model, of the anatomical part which had been healed.

While the cult of Aesculapius fluctuated about AD 300, the concept of miracle cures still remains through the sanction of miracles by the Roman Catholic church. The collection of crutches left behind by the sick and disabled at Lourdes presents a similar scene to an Aesculapian temple; the miracle was achieved through prayer rather than dreams.

Aristotle wrote that a miracle is contrary to nature, but not contrary to nature as a whole; rather, contrary to it as it appears in most cases. For in regard to the eternal nature which acts with necessity, nothing comes to being contrary with it. In other words, miracles are events whose causes are unknown; therefore, miracles need not be excluded from a concept of science in medicine. The Greeks felt this need present no contradiction by being beyond experience. To be opposed to miracles is to assume that nothing can happen without intelligent reason.

The idea of disease as a punishment for sin originated in the early Semitic civilizations of the Middle East. Disease came to be seen as a tribulation to be borne, and it became the duty of the citizen to help the sick to bear their punishment. Hebrew medicine, although influenced by neighbouring cultures and thought, relied on the Talmud for guidance, rather than on any systematic medical texts. The Hebrews believed that one God was the source of health and illness. In the Old Testament, there are several expressions of such a nature, for example, 'I will put none of these diseases on thee... for I am the Lord, that healeth thee' (Exodus 15:26). Anatomical knowledge was more advanced than elsewhere, owing to the dissection of sacrificial animals; however, Hebrew physicians were also priests who could appeal to God on behalf of the supplicant. When lay physicians were introduced they came to have jurisdiction over internal conditions; but demons were still believed to cause the more obscure conditions such as epilepsy, asthma or mental illness. However, the supreme controlling force who sent the demons was still the Supreme Being. For example, in the first book of Samuel, Saul's mental illness is described as being caused by an evil spirit sent from the Lord.

Illness for the Greeks also held a connotation of sin. Not that illness was God's punishment so much that the patient had sinned against Nature — which demanded a reciprocal relationship. The Greeks used the term 'eukrasia' which literally translates as 'the state of being well mixed' or well. The opposite term is 'dyskrasia' or a 'state of being ill mixed' or sick. It was through conserving symmetry in the different spheres of his life that an individual protected his health, and it was by teaching his patients how to conserve and restore it that physicians such as Hippocrates made themselves indispensable. Consequently, the Greek physician had to be an ethical instructor, as well as a curer of bodily diseases (Bürgel 1976).

The healing of the sick played such an important part in all religious cults at the time of Christ that the new religion probably could not have successfully competed with the old unless it also held some promise of miraculous healing (Sigerist 1962). Christianity came into the world as a religion of healing.

The concept of a 'soul' also pre-dated Christianity. The obvious connection between air and life had not escaped the Greeks, for without it animal matter could not live nor could fire be sustained. So vital air, or *pneuma*, became associated with ideas of life and motion, and led to a century's search for its special element which we now know as oxygen (Jones 1947). Aristotle held that the *pneuma* was related to the soul. The soul was said to be composed of special light and smooth atoms similar to those of fire, but not identical (Phillips 1973). The special location of these soul atoms was in the head, but they could travel through the body to give life. It was believed that these atoms were always attempting to leave the body under pressure from atoms outside it, but since all air contained many of these atoms they were replaced in respiration. Death occurred when the pressure from outside became too great and respiration ceased, causing the soul atoms to flow out.

Roman and Arabic civilizations

In the Roman empire, magic, religion and medicine became so intertwined as to be indistinguishable. Medicine to the Romans was but, 'a specialized segment of generalized concepts in philosophy and tradition, given organization and effectiveness by collections of observations in encyclopaedic form' (Scarborough 1969). Rome gradually turned from the natural answers, posed in Greek heritage of questioning, to the mystical all-encompassing solutions of religion. The poet Horace wrote, 'the words of the wise on magic charms you can use, to sooth the pain and practically rout the disease'.

The Roman physician Galen, born about AD 129, produced the most complete medical 'encyclopaedia' of the classical era. Not much was added to his work until the sixteenth century. Galen believed in the Platonic doctrine of three 'souls' that ruled the body. These souls 'lived' in the heart, brain and liver, and he named them choleric, rational and sensual souls. He also believed in the Greek humours, in *pneuma*, and that astrology could have some effect on health.

The medical approach of Greek physicians, such as Hippocrates, and Roman physicians such as Galen, can be summed up as being ecological in viewpoint and persuasion — ecology being the science of relation of things (Galdston 1981). Such concepts survived the collapse and disintegration of the Roman empire and prevailed until the advent of the Renaissance in the sixteenth century.

In Europe, Arabic (or Islamic) medicine took over from Rome as the dominant influence and reached its peak in the ninth and tenth centuries. Influenced by Greek ideas, the Islamic physician, or *hakim*, layed emphasis on an individual cure. Many Arabic rulers were also physicians, and hospitals were adopted from the Hindus as an intrinsic part of the Islamic medical system (Basham 1976). Despite the prominence of physicians such as Rhazes (who died in AD 925) Arabic influence declined, because authority shifted from the physician to the Prophet (Mohammed) and from reason to religious belief. Medicine was administered to the patient not because it was known to cure, but because the Prophet approved of it (Bürgel 1976).

Oriental civilizations

Arabic medicine was also strongly influenced by Indian traditions, which reached their classical form at the onset of the Christian era. The science of medicine in India was known as '*āgurveda*' or 'the science of (living to a ripe) age' (Basham 1976). The Indian philosophy emphasized means of preserving health, rather than curing disease. Life and health in each individual were controlled, in part, by his 'karma' or destiny, or by the effect of good and evil deeds done in former lives, and by efforts and conduct in the present.

The archetypal Indian physician was the divine sage or *vaidya*. His aims were not only curative but preventive; to manage the whole life of his client and help prolong it. Health was thought to be conditioned by the balance of three primary elements — wind, gall, and mucus. Hindu medicine maintained that natural law governed the body, and that man afflicted himself, rather than divine intervention. This placed emphasis on a mixture of nutritional and physical therapies. For example, the eating of 'hot' and 'cold' food to promote 'balance' in the body is still practised today.

The *vaidya* was assisted in his work by trained nurses, normally referred to in the masculine, *paricāraka*. Nursing appears to have been a definite trade or profession in early India, and not merely a task to be performed by any domestic servant. Hol (1948) claimed that the ideal qualities of a nurse at this time were 'to be devoted and friendly, untiringly watchful, not inclined to disgust, and knowledgeable enough to fulfill the orders of the doctor'. In Graeco-Roman society the sick tended to be cared for at home. Where skilled nursing was called for, and the client wealthy, the Greek physician often left one of his pupils in charge. For the less important, slaves and women did the nursing.

Although individual behaviour and health were perceived as being related, in India epidemic diseases such as cholera were thought to be caused by Hindu disease goddesses. The function of such a goddess was — and in some areas still remains — to punish communities that become sinful, by bringing disease, crop failure and loss of livestock. To the extent that punishment is not intended, or that appropriate strategies are adopted to remove sin, the same goddesses may be regarded as protective figures who prevent misfortune (Beales 1976).

Indian medicine was influenced in its turn by Chinese traditions and beliefs. Traditional Chinese medicine did not develop from any knowledge of anatomy, physiology, or biochemistry, but rather as an inductive science through defining the relationship between different functions aimed at finding the value or quality of a relationship (Pokert 1976). The basic standards of such value comprise the polar combinations of 'Yin' and 'Yang'. 'Yang' implies all that is structured, responsive, conservative and positive, while 'Yin' corresponds to all that is active, competitive, negative and aggressive. Once again, the aim of the healer was to achieve balance or harmony within the individual. If a man became too aggressive, angry or envious, he created disharmony both within himself and in the Universe.

For centuries, China was dominated by Confucian philosophy, which was concerned primarily with social ethics; that is, the relation of the individual to a hierarchical society. In the Confucian social pyramid the physician held a low status, and the boundaries of society were so fixed that proficiency in medicine rarely procured any official honour. Medical enquiry had to rely on the complementary philosophy of Taoism. Up to the thirteenth century, Taoism carried connotations of priestly or shamanistic functions (Pokert 1976). Consequently, a Taoist/medical man could transcend the social barriers in China by studying what society considered of little consequence — a type of medical dilettante. The Confucian straightjacket meant that the Chinese medical tradition made little progress from the fourteenth century.

Similar concepts, involving cosmological and individual harmony, are also expressed in Japanese traditional medicine. It is based on the concept of '*ki*' which has been defined as 'the essence which sustains the body'. Hashimoto (1966) claimed that 'this essence has a mysterious power which works invisibly, and which exists within everything in the universe'. When adversely affected, a Japanese was likely to try to restore this balance with nature through taking traditional medicine, resting in bed, bathing in hot springs, massage or acupuncture.

Greek and Arab physicians were also aware of the influence a man's belief had on the state of the body, and on the success or failure of therapeutic measures. They recognized that any approach was useful if the patient believed in it. Acquiring the confidence of the patient was regarded as a vital factor in the process of healing. Arab physicians, for example, were advised to wear white, well-scented clothing, to have hair and nails of moderate length, to proceed to the bedside at a moderate speed, and not to harangue the patient with unnecessary questions (Bürgel 1976).

The importance of psychology was carried into the recognition of psychosomatic disorders. Drugs and music were recommended for depressive states; however, chains and whipping were often used for various psychotic disorders.

The re-emergence of European medicine

European medicine was revived at Salerno, in Italy, in the late tenth century through the establishing of a university course in medicine. A second centre was established in the eleventh century, at Avicenna, and other European universities emerged from the fourteenth century. However, this form of revival restricted the teaching and practice of medicine to certain centres, with a consequent decrease in the numbers of roaming physicians who went wherever the demand was. In addition, women were excluded from university, and those interested in healing either continued to practise traditional medicine or entered religious orders. The centralization of medicine allowed further restriction of entry through State legislation and State-governed formal examinations. Traditional medicine, and its practitioners, came to be regarded with suspicion. Szasz (1971) claimed that, 'because the mediaeval church, with the support of kings, princes, and secular authorities, controlled medical education and practice, the witch hunts constitute, among other things, an early instance of the "professional" repudiating the skills, and interfering with, the rights of the "non-professional" to minister to the person'.

Thomas (1971) claimed that fear of witchcraft, in Britain, was also related to the social tensions of emerging capitalism. People felt powerless in the face of illness and death and the economic and social antagonism, not justifiable in experience, were attributed to sorcery. Outside areas of European influence traditional medicine, and healers, continued to be perceived as a valuable health care resource and even today continue as a popular alternative, or supplement, to Westernized medicine, often with State support.

Admittedly, this does not contribute evidence for the value of medicine in biological terms, but it does indicate some adaptive value in the supportive or psychosocial sense. European medicine appeared to lose this supportive value by the institutionalization of medicine in the medieval period, through religious dogma, to the detriment of total health care. Galdston (1981) claimed that 'ridgified in a system of formulas and dominated by mysticism, medicine was forced to exist in a state of scholastic dogmatism in which it is difficult to find any animatory ideas'. Magic rituals and traditional medical systems became resuscitated in Christian theological forms. When a person became sick he addressed himself to God. Often a confession of sin was demanded of him. Hepworth and Turner (1982) claimed that 'A confession is not only an admission of guilt, it is a recognition of the concept of guilt and the right of the (religious) authorities to define misdemeanour and remorse'. The reward for confessing, and the element of forgiveness it induces, reinforces, in part, the rightness of the prevailing order. There is little evidence directly comparing Christians with non-Christians on measures of guilt, but what does exist suggests that the former tend to have more intense feelings of guilt (Peretti 1969).

Intermediaries to the Almighty were often used — for example, the Virgin Mary to whose healing intervention over forty churches were dedicated in France alone (including Lourdes). Saints also became identified with· various diseases and were approached in prayer for intervention. For example, St Vitus for epileptics, St Anthony for ergotism, St Sebastian for plague, and St Blaise for throat disorders. Relics of saints were said to hold miraculous powers, and medals and portraits began to replace amulets and talismans. This led to the evolution of the pilgrimage for prophylactic or penitential advantage. The modern hospital system had its origins in the sheltering of such large numbers of pilgrims, whether sick or well. Nursing the sick, as a Christian duty, found a natural base in monastic orders. However, according to Michelet (1937), the Church had little to offer the suffering peasantry at this time except to claim that sickness was an affliction of God for sin, and if endured would reduce suffering in the life to come. The glorification of suffering depends partly on belief in predestination or determinism, one of the speculative consequences of which is to diminish any secondary causes of disease. The medieval argument centred on there being no such thing as natural causality, even in the absence of microbiological evidence; that all phenomena are immediately introduced by the prime cause — namely God. This attitude demanded a total and passive reliance on the Almighty, and often denied any role for medical teaching. The physician had to counteract such dogma by claiming that if God was responsible for inflicting the disease, he must also be responsible for the provision of the cure.

Traditional values in modern medicine

The basis for traditional or folk medicine is that the body and mind are indivisibly linked. A morbid somatic condition is not something entirely objective and outside of the consciousness of the patient. The condition may or may not be cured according to the accuracy of the diagnosis and the precision of surgery or chemotherapy. The conscious understanding and efforts of the patient, his family and friends, are critical factors in the therapeutic process. Jones (1965) claimed that 'the greatest sin against the human spirit is closure against the diversity and variety of experience — a narrow dogmatism that insists on the absolute and exclusive validity of some particular language, and the particular version of reality that this language articulates'.

The pattern of the emergence of medicine from the nineteenth century led to the belief that all medical knowledge and skill be determined solely by the laws of mathematics and logic, in order to secure recognition for medicine, through making everything permanent and absolute. However, health is a state of perception and experience, and not merely the absence of one or other disease entity. When the correlates of a person's perception of their own health are examined, the presence or absence of psychological and spiritual distress are major predictors of how the person feels about himself.

Critical rationalism has led many individuals in the twentieth century to identify themselves almost exclusively with their conscious image of themselves, so that they come to believe what they know about themselves from past experience. Yet such knowledge about self can be very limited. (Jung 1972) claimed that our concepts of time and space have only approximate validity, and there is a wide field for minor or major deviance. In illness, this partially complete picture of the world, and the individual's part in it, becomes disrupted. As time and space take on different relativities, in the new situation, a different or additional dimension is needed to give support and allow reconstruction to take place. For example, many people have a need to maintain the assumption that life will have an indefinite continuity beyond present existence. By such belief they live more sensibly, feel happier and are more at peace with themselves and others.

While individual nurses have always recognized the multidimensional components of health and illness, the institutions of nursing have been constructed within the medical model. However, nursing cannot be reduced to an absolute science, because nurses are essentially humanistic, and through their prolonged contact with the patient they can never come to deny this. The distinguishing characteristics of humanism include adopting a wide perspective, being willing to wait patiently for results, attempting to reconcile divergence and holding hope in the educability of mankind (Galdston 1981). The Humanist is an individual with a keen social conscience, but one who is under no illusion that he has to function in far from ideal situations. Humanism imbibes a recognition that the patient is both everyman, in that he shares characteristics with all other human beings; and a single individual, in that he is different in ability and need from all others.

While medicine has pursued a doctrine of 'great men, great discoveries', nursing has always been concerned with the promotion of total physical, social and spiritual well-being of individuals, and not merely with the conquest of disease. Bellamy (1983) claimed that the dominant medical model has created a perception of man as isolated and dependent, while the process of nursing sets man in a much wider context suggesting corporate roots of health and illness.

The care each person receives, therefore, should rest on measuring particular considerations against his universal needs. Most hospital wards, however, continue to be run on the theme of utilitarianism, that is 'the greatest good for the greatest number'. The fewer the resources the greater this philosophy, and the more likely it will be that dehumanization will occur. Dehumanization is essentially an unequal and imperfect recognition of the quality of human personality (Mechanic 1968). The spiritual needs of the patient contain elements of both the individual and the universal. While the universal can be sustained the individual spiritual need can become, as well as the physical, subsumed in the socialization of the institution.

Occasionally, the human race as a whole appears to waken to a profound moral crisis, the predisposition of which is often obscure. At such times, the usual economic or ethical frameworks of society appear to be defective, and the norms and values by which Man has grown accustomed to measure the worth of things becomes invalid. Each individual, when faced by sudden illness or disability, is likely to undergo a similar moral crisis. Previous experience may fail him, as he seeks explanation or reason for his hazardous situation. He tries to regain the equilibrium and harmony of wellness. Where a modern physician can offer little help the patient's search may lead him to turn to alternative medicine, such as acupuncture, hypnosis, osteopathy, or herbal cures; some of which have acquired varying degrees of recognition by authoritative medicine in recent years. But for his spiritual well-being, the alternatives to authoritative religion are more restricted. An approach to a faith healer, for instance, would be viewed with greater consternation than an approach to an osteopath. Is a minister of religion ever invited to accompany a consultant on ward rounds? What would be the reaction of hospital staff if a faith healer visited the ward? While most doctors and nurses will accept, albeit at times reluctantly, that there is a role for alternative medicine, the value of an alternative spiritual aid to formal religion is rarely, if ever discussed. Yet what is needed in health care is a greater awareness that the spiritual needs of human beings are manifold and cannot be simply categorized into a nursing card index 'RC', 'Prot', or 'Jew'. The ancients learned this lesson well; they listened to the patient, and adapted their spiritual care to what the patient wanted. Spiritual management is no less relevant today than it was centuries ago, but this appears to be a lesson that we are having to relearn.

References

Alexander F G and Selesnick S T (1966) The history of Psychiatry: an Evaluation of Psychiatric Thought and Practice from Prehistoric Times to the Present, Mentor Books

Basham A L (1976) The practice of medicine in Ancient and mediaeval India, in C Leslie (Editor) Asian Medical Systems, a Comparative Study, University of California Press

Beales A (1976) Curers in South India, in C Leslie (Editor) Asian Medical Systems, a Comparative Study, University of California Press

Bellamy P C W (1983) The nursing process : a problem of practical theology, Nursing Times, Occasional Papers, 79: 35–36

Bürgel J C (1976) Secular and religious features of mediaeval Arabic medicine in C Leslie (Editor) Asian Medical Systems, a Comparative Study, University of California Press

Galdston I (1981) Social and Historical Foundations of Modern Medicine, Brunner-Mazel

Hashimoto M (1966) Japanese Acupuncture, Garden City Press

Hepworth M and Turner B S (1982) Confession: Studies in Deviance and Religion, Routledge and Kegan Paul

Hol Z (1948) Hindu Medicine, Johns Hopkins University Press

Jones W H S (1947) The Medical Writings of Anonymous Londinensis, Cambridge University Press

Jones W T (1965) The Sciencies and Humanities: Conflict and Reconciliation, University of California Press

Jung C G (1972) Memories, Dreams, Reflections, Fontana Books

Kemp P (1935) Healing Ritual, Faber and Faber

Mechanic D (1968) Medical Sociology, Free Press

Michelet, J (1937) Satanism and Witchcraft, The Citadel Press

Osler, Sir W (1948) Aequanimatas, H K Lewis

Peretti, P O (1969) Guilt in moral development: a comparative study, Psychological Reports, 25: 739–745

Phillips, E D (1973) Greek Medicine, Thames and Hudson

Pokert, M (1976) The intellectual and social impulses behind the evolution of traditional Chinese medicine, in C Leslie (Editor) Asian Medical Systems: a Comparative Study, University of California Press

Scarborough, J (1969) Roman Medicine, Thames and Hudson

Sigerist, H E (1962) Civilization and Disease, Phoenix Books

Szasz, T (1971) The Manufacture of Madness, Delta Books

Temkin, O and Temkin, C L (Editors) (1967) Ancient Medicine: Selected Papers of Ludwig Edelstein, Johns Hopkins Press

Thomas, K (1971) Religion and the Decline of Magic, Weidenfeld and Nicholson

CHAPTER 2

RELIGIOUS BELIEFS, PRACTICES AND PHILOSOPHIES

Introduction

There have been many definitions of religion. Some authorities define it as man's effort to achieve the highest possible good, by adjusting his way of life to an ideal power, and a belief in that power, usually termed 'God'. Some define it as a saving relationship between man and one or more gods, or supernatural beings. For others, religion may be a way of living rather than a way of believing. For our purposes, however, it is sufficient to state that man seems to have a need to relate to what Talcott Parsons termed 'transcendental reference'; that religion, although concerned with something beyond the observable events of everyday existence, is important and not peripheral to the everyday business of human activity; that man's relation to and his attitude toward the 'beyond' may have practical implications for his acceptance of certain basic characteristics of the human condition. Religion helps man answer basic questions about life and death, and the unexplained happenings in the world around him.

This chapter offers an overview of the beliefs and practices of the world's major religions and attempts to identify a few of their common features. Although it is accepted that not all members of any particular religious group will equally adhere to the beliefs and practices of their religion, the chapter takes a conservative stance. It does not attempt to give anything like a coverage of the facts relevant to any group, but serves to illustrate the importance of religious beliefs, practices and other philosophies for thousands of millions of people, and thereby for the great majority of our patients.

The major religions

The major religions practised in the world today are: Judaism, Christianity, Islam, Hinduism, Buddhism, Jainism, Sikhism, Confucianism, Taoism, Shinto and Zoroastrianism. Each of these holds within it various groups, or denominations, that tend to lay emphasis on different aspects of the parent religion. All the major religions have basic traditions, beliefs and practices.

Judaism

The Jewish Faith, Judaism, is the oldest religion of the western world and was one of the first religions to teach belief in one God (monotheism). Jews believe in one God who is good and just and demands righteous conduct. 'I will show thee, O man, what is good, and what the Lord requireth of thee: verily, to do judgement, and to love mercy, and to walk solicitous with thy God' (Micah 6:8). The Jewish Faith centres around this belief.

Tradition teaches that Abraham, considered by many as the father of the Jewish people, made an agreement promising to worship God and to spread His Word. And when a Jewish boy is 8 days old he is circumcised as a symbol of this 'covenant' God made with Abraham. However, the Jewish religion probably began when God's law was given to Moses and the Israelite people (Exodus 20:1–17). Judaism is founded on the laws and teachings of the Hebrew Bible, or Old Testament — the Torah, the Prophets, and the Writings — and of the Talmud.

The Torah serves as the religious structure of Judaism containing the Ten Commandments and the basic laws; it consists of the first five books of the Bible (the Five Books of Moses). The Prophets tells about the Jews in Canaan, the kingdoms of Judah and Israel and the Babylonian Exile; it includes the teachings of such prophets as Isaiah, Amos and Micah. The Writings includes proverbs and psalms. The Talmud (an interpretation by Rabbis and scholars of Biblical law in order to adapt it to daily life) serves as a guide to the civil laws, religious laws and teachings of Judaism.

There are about 13 million Jews and the religion has three main groups: Orthodox, Conservative, and Reform; but faith in one God forms the basis of Judaism: 'Hear O Israel, the Lord our God, the Lord is One' (Deuteronomy 6:4). Jews believe that God created man in His own image (Genesis 5:1) and that all men deserve to be treated with dignity and respect; they stress the importance of freedom and ethical conduct in the world. Orthodox Jews still await a personal Messiah to redeem mankind on earth. Conservative and Reform Jews believe that freedom and peace will come with God's help and the efforts of all men.

Christianity and Islam are both derived from Judaism. Both religions accept the belief in one God and the ethical teachings of the Hebrew Bible.

Christianity

The Christian religion began with a movement of Jews in Palestine who believed that Jesus of Nazareth was the Saviour for whom the people had been waiting. They called Jesus the *Christ* or *Messiah* — the promised deliverer of the Jews — and became known as Christians. They followed Jesus around the country to listen to him instruct and preach about the Kingdom of God, and watched him perform miracles. Jesus (like the Old Testament prophets) demanded justice toward men and humility toward God. He also preached mercy, stressed brotherly love and told of the love of God for all.

The Jewish religious leaders of the time of Christ considered his claim — that he was the promised deliverer of the Jews — to be blasphemous, and the Roman leaders believed that his claim to be King of the Jews amounted to treason and might cause an uprising against Roman rule in Palestine. As a result Jesus was tried and condemned to death. He was crucified on Good Friday.

The death of Christ caused his followers (disciples) to be frightened and disillusioned; they scattered across the country and went into hiding. However, the news that Jesus was reported alive on the first Easter morning brought them together again and, since then, Christianity has become the largest of the world's religious groups. There are over a billion Christians, about 600 million of whom are Roman Catholic; 270 million are Protestant (of different denominations) and 150 million Eastern Orthodox.

Thus Christian beliefs and practices belong to the teachings and life of Jesus Christ, as written in the New Testament, and to the Hebrew Bible (or Old Testament). The various Christian groups tend to lay emphasis on different aspects of Christ's teachings, but the main themes stress God's love for all and that Christians should love God and their neighbour. 'Thou shalt love the Lord thy God with all thy heart, and with all thy soul, and with all thy strength, and with all thy mind; and thy neighbour as thyself' (Luke 10:27). The 'Rising from the Dead' on Easter Sunday is called the Resurrection and forms one of the fundamental beliefs of Christianity. Followers of the Christian faith accept that the death of Jesus Christ reconciled mankind to God and that, by his resurrection, he overcame death and evil; and that those who are good Christians will experience this new life beyond the grave.

Islam

The Islam religion began with the preaching of Mohammed in Mecca about 600 years after the birth of Christianity. Mohammed taught that he was a prophet sent to call his people to worship Allah (God). Before Mohammed's teachings, the Arabs worshipped many gods and obvious injustices of life happened in Mecca. The new prophet preached the punishment of evil-doers; that there is only one God and that he, Mohammed, was God's messenger. Followers of the teachings of Mohammed are called Moslems.

The revelations of Mohammed form the Koran (the Sacred book of the Moslems), parts of which resemble the Bible, the Apocrypha and the Talmud. The Koran holds many stories about the prophets that appear in the Hebrew Bible and also contains stories about Jesus of Nazareth. Islam, built upon Judaism and Christianity, claims to be the Faith to which these religions led. Moslems believe that Mohammed was the last of the prophets; that Jesus and the prophets of the Hebrew Bible were Mohammed's predecessors.

The Koran, like the Bible (Old and New Testaments), stresses ethics and morals and teaches virtue and justice. Their religion teaches Moslems that life on earth prepares man for the life to come; that there is a life after death in heaven or in hell. Moslems believe that death leads to everlasting life and that there is a last day, or day of judgement, when God's justice will be made known. Everyone will receive the record — kept by the angels — of earthly deeds and the good will go to heaven and the wicked to hell.

Islam, like Judaism and Christianity, teaches its followers to believe in the absolute unity and power of a just and merciful Creator of the whole universe. The word Islam is usually taken to mean 'peace through submission to Allah', and the Faith requires that man repent and cleanse himself on earth so that he can attain heaven after death.

Islam, one of the world's largest religions (about a half a billion followers) has two main groups: Sunnites and Shiites; there have also been a number of smaller groups, for example, the Wahabis are strong in Saudi Arabia. Most Moslems are Sunnites; the Baha'i Faith grew out of the Shiite group.

Hinduism

Unlike Judaism or Christianity or Islam, Hinduism — the dominant religion of India — has no historical founder; it claims no single prophet or messiah. According to tradition, the *Laws of the Vedas*, representing the period of early worship, were revealed to *rishis* (spiritual men) about 1000 BC. The word Hindu comes from the Persian *hind:* the name for the River Indus region of northern India.

The religion teaches that Brahman is the Supreme Spirit; perfect and unchanging and above human description. Hinduism teaches that only permanent is real and only Brahman, the essence of every living thing, is real. Thus, because every creature has a soul which comes from the Supreme Soul, Hindus respect all life. For example, as a symbol of Man's identity with all life, Hindus consider the cow sacred.

Hinduism emphasizes the one absolute, infinite Brahman but allows worship of many other gods as ways of understanding the indescribable neuter Brahman. Examples of such gods are Brahma (the Creator), Siva (the Destroyer) and Vishnu (the Preserver or Renewer or god of Love); Hindus pay special heed to Rama and Krishna — two of the greatest forms of Vishnu — and their religion holds that these and other gods are only different aspects of the one Brahman.

The ultimate aim of man's soul is union with Brahman but this cannot be achieved in one lifetime. According to the *Law of Karma*, a person's actions in one life determine the next life he will lead. Hinduism teaches reincarnation or transmigration of the soul and that the soul is freed, from the cycles of birth and death, when it attains union with Brahman. The *Bhagavadgita*, the most esteemed book of Hinduism, stresses the importance of deed, thought and faith as the ways of reaching Brahman; yoga —the discipline of mind and body — is the enabler.

Hinduism recognized a caste or hereditary social order and the teachings of reincarnation and Karma were used to justify the place and rank of each person. Untouchability was outlawed in the late 1940s.

The Hindu religion, with a following of over 400 million, has given rise to many sects. Yet almost all of its sects continue to believe in the doctrines of reincarnation and Karma. Buddhism stemmed from Hinduism and Sikhism is a blend of Hinduism and Islam.

Buddhism

Buddhism stemmed from Hinduism about 2500 years ago. It was founded by Siddhartha Gautama (a Hindu prince) who became known as Gautama Buddha. The word Buddha means 'Fully Enlightened or Awakened One'.

Siddhartha Gautama the son of a rajah was born about 560 BC at Kapilavasta; a town in what is now Nepal. As a young man Gautama was concerned about the miseries of life in India and felt a strong desire to help his people find happiness. He gave up his own riches and lifestyle, and set out to search for the truth which would bring peace and happiness to sufferers. Gautama discovered the answer (the Four Noble Truths) as he sat on a river bank under a sacred fig tree. He then was called Buddha.

The first Noble Truth is that suffering and human existence, or way of life, are strongly linked. This led to Gautama believing (the second Truth) that suffering is caused by human desire for pleasure; a desire which impedes knowledge and insight. Gautama believed that desire should be for goodness — not evil. The third Truth is that man will become free from sorrow by destroying evil desire. And the fourth Truth (the Noble Eightfold Path) teaches that right belief, aspiration, speech, action, livelihood, effort, thought and meditation will lead to the end of the state of suffering. Gautama termed this ideal state (of perfect freedom and passionless peace) Nirvana; not a heaven, as Christians generally think of heaven, but a state of quality of mind.

Buddha stressed the importance of knowing one's self to prevent self-centredness, desire, disappointment and sorrow. He taught that this knowledge of self could happen through self-control, humility, generosity and mercy; that man must reject anger, passion and sin. He also stressed love as a virtue and the importance of loving one's enemies. Gautama's most devoted disciples formed a monastic order because the ideal could be attained only after thorough training in a monastery. He also had lay followers who could stay with their friends and possessions but could not kill or steal, be unchaste, lie, or take strong drink — in order to achieve a higher rebirth on earth. Buddhism also believes in reincarnation.

The religion began in India and helped break down the problems of caste by uniting many people. It slowly disappeared from India (about AD 1000) but spread to Tibet, China, Japan and south-eastern Asia. The two main sects are the Hinayana and the Mahayana. The former has maintained the teachings of Gautama. The Mahayana believes that there are many buddhas and has a doctrine of heaven and hell with salvation by faith and grace. Tibetan Buddhism (Lamaism) is a form of Mahayana. The total number of Buddhists is about 220 million, and most of them live in China.

Jainism

Jainism, like Buddhism, is an outgrowth of Hinduism founded in India (by Mahavira) about 2500 years ago. Jains (conquerors) do not worship any particular god, they practise asceticism to conquer the desires of the body and believe in transmigration of the soul; after the soul has inhabited many bodies it becomes free and peaceful. The religion teaches non-violence and stresses love and kindness. Jains are forbidden to kill or injure any living organism — even the insect is sacred. The total number of Jains is about 2 million and almost all of them live in India.

Sikhism

Sikhism is a religion of the Punjab region of north-western India. The word Sikh means 'disciple'. Founded by Guru Nanak (about 400 years ago) as a means of uniting Moslems and all castes of Hindus into one fraternity, it combines elements of Islam and Hinduism. Guru Nanak accepted the Islam teaching that there is one just and merciful Creator of the whole universe, and believed that every person should have direct communication with God. He taught ethics and morals and that no person should have special privileges by reason of, for example, birth or sex. Sikhism also accepted doctrines of Hinduism such as transmigration of the soul; that the soul is reborn into many bodies before it is pure enough to be united with the infinite Supreme Spirit.

Followers of modern Sikhism should wear: uncut hair *(Keshas);* the comb *(Kanga)* to keep the hair in place under a turban; the steel bangle *(Kara)* to remind them of the unity of God and their religious obligations; the short sword *(Kirpan)* — usually worn as a brooch or pin — to symbolize defence and dignity, and under-shorts *(Kachcha)* to remind of sexual principles.

Although many followers of Sikhism are farmers, the religion has a strong military and political history. Sikhs built up their military power to protect them against Moslems and other religious groups. They were defeated by the British in the mid-1800s but supported the British in the first and second World Wars. And in 1966 — to satisfy the Sikhs — the Indian government created a separate State where Punjabi is spoken in the Punjab region. The central shrine of the religion is at Amritsar (in the Indian Punjab) where the Sacred Book — *Ad Granth* — is read aloud every day. There are almost 8 million Sikhs in India.

Confucianism

Confucianism is one of the principle religions of China. The other major religions are Buddhism and Taoism; Islam is important for minority peoples. Christianity has a relatively small number of followers.

Confucianism was founded by Confucius (a wise man) about 2500 years ago. His ambition was to enable people to develop a moral sense of responsibility toward each other. He taught that men should be gentle and kind to each other and show respect to older people and superiors. His followers emphasize specific duties and behaviours of five basic relation-ships : ruler and subject, father and son, husband and wife, elder and younger brother, and friend and friend. Thus many authorities see Confucianism as a system of ethics rather than a religion, but Confucianism also has a religious attitude. Confucius believed in a Supreme Being *(Shang Ti)* and stressed the importance of traditional practices of Chinese religion. He aimed to restore the beliefs and practices of the prophet emperors and wise men of the past; China has a history (in written form) that goes back about 3500 years.

In short, Confucianism stresses loyalty and harmony within the family, traditional worship and obedience to the authority of society. Confucianists believe that something in man survives bodily death even though the human cannot understand how. The *Five Classics* offer the teachings of Confucius to about 300 million followers.

Taoism

Tradition holds that Taoism belongs to the teachings of Lao-Tse (the old master) who lived in China about 2500 years ago. The name of the religion derives from Lao-Tse's book, *Tao Te Ching (The Way and Its Power)*, which is the Sacred Book of Taoism. Tao means 'the way' and followers of the religion believe that 'the way' of life is close harmony with nature, and that man has caused disharmony by substituting the ordered and harmonic way with his own designs. Followers accept that Tao is the ruler of heaven; heaven rules earth and earth rules its people. Taoists believe that man can find peace and happiness only by seeking to restore harmony through simplicity and humility. They stress the need to worship Tao and to be good to all things while avoiding distinction and honour for themselves.

Taoists, like Confucianists, believe that something in man survives bodily death. The religion includes much magic and superstition; it has about 30 million followers in China.

Shinto

Shinto, meaning the 'Way of the Gods' is the original religion of Japan. The other major religions in Japan are Buddhism, Confucianism, Taoism and Christianity.

The religion dates back to the origins of Japanese civilization (about 2500 years ago) when the people worshipped the spirits of nature. The highest god of Shintoism was the sun. Shintoists also worshipped spirits of the forests, rivers and seas; numbers of followers still worship such deities. Alongside this, the Japanese hold a strong loyalty to their history and Shintoism accommodated ancestor worship. Confucianistic thought played a part in raising ethical standards in Shinto, and Buddhism influenced Shinto philosophy.

The religion grew into two main groups; Sect Shinto and State Shinto (of the 1870s). In the former, individual sects use the teachings of a particular leader to construct programmes of education and worship. State Shinto, which developed to promote patriotism around the emperor, taught its followers that the emperor was descended from the Sun Goddess and should be worshipped as a god. The government supported State Shinto until after the Second World War. The Emperor Hirohito denied his divinity at that time; the government and emperor abandoned State Shinto in 1947.

About 80 million Japanese still follow Sect Shinto (there are about 80 000 shrines and temples); many of them also practise Buddhism.

Zoroastrianism

Zoroastrianism, an ancient religion, was founded by a Persian prophet Zoroaster (about 600 BC), who believed in the one and only god Ahura-Mazda and taught that people will merit eternal life in paradise by helping Ahura-Mazda fight the powers of evil. Zoroaster believed that even the most evil people attain salvation; that the good go directly to heaven and the wicked go to heaven after purification in hell.

The six names of their god (Ahura-Mazda) help to illustrate Zoroastrianism thought. The god is called: the Good Thought; the Beauty of Holiness; Righteousness; Perfect Health; Dominion and Immortality. Zoroastrians accept that the greatest virtues are good thoughts, words and deeds; the greatest evil is the lie. The Holy Book of Zoroastrianism is the *Zend-Avesta* which praises the powers of nature as well as Zoroaster's one and only god. There are about 100 000 Zoroastrins (Parsis) in the world today and most of them live in the Bombay region of India. The religion has a number of small sects.

Common features of the major religions

All of the major religions (outlined above) strive to achieve the highest possible good by teaching their followers to believe in an ideal standard or Supreme Being. Most of the religions teach about one pure Supreme Spirit — usually termed God — and accept their god as just and all powerful and the Creator of the universe. Believers are required to adjust their ways of life to become pure enough to be united with the Supreme Spirit. Most religions accept that there is a presence in man that survives death of the body. Some teach that man will meet his judgement after death and be sent to heaven or hell. Certain religions teach reincarnation before union with the Supreme Spirit, while others are unsure about life after death but generally accept that something in man endures beyond death.

Every religion has a set of doctrines and code of behaviour found in sacred book/s. And educated men (ministers, priests and rabbis, for example) receive extensive training to teach the laws and codes of their religion. Some religions are very definite about how their believers should act toward God. For example, many are required to worship one god only — and not to worship idols — and how to pray; Moslems are required to pray five times every day.. Many religions use symbols and ceremonies to aid worship. Symbols are reminders of teachings and reinforcers of beliefs. The cross, to symbolize the crucifixion of Jesus Christ, reminds Christians of Christ's sacrifice, and his love of all men, and the good need to love and make allowances for others. Ceremonies help worship through action (mostly shared with others) and presentation or display. Genuflecting, kneeling, praying aloud with others, hymn singing, lighted candles held aloft in a procession, colourful garments, and so on allow believers to express their feelings for God in an open and satisfying way. Ceremonies usually occur on fixed days (Holy Days) and usually happen in places of worship — churches, mosques, synagogues and temples, for example — but need not be confined to any time or place.

Followers of almost every religion are required to exercise the teachings of their religion in a personal manner, and most are taught that things such as murder, stealing, adultery, unchaste behaviour and dishonesty are evil. All the major religions condemn selfishness, teach love and stress the importance of not hurting other people. Beyond these common codes of conduct, certain religious teachings are designed to influence everyday aspects of a believer's way of life. Followers of Asian religions are extremely embarrassed when undressing in the company of strangers, and consider cleanliness to be very important. For example, many Asians will prefer to shower because they dislike sitting in their own dirty bath water, and may dislike having to touch unclean material with the right hand; the left hand is normally used for such things as personal toilet while the right hand is used for eating and clean tasks. Followers of certain religions abhor any form of mutilation and some are particularly sensitive about killing. Jains are forbidden to kill any living organism and will even wear masks to prevent accidentally inhaling and killing insect life. Hindus are not allowed to eat beef and many Buddhists are vegetarian. Jews are forbidden to eat pork or to combine meat and milk at any one meal. These are just a few of the sensitivities carried by followers of the many different religions. A wide range of beliefs and practices accompany every religion and these extend far beyond the scope of this chapter. It is sufficient to state that the proper management of intimate relations with believers, especially believers who are ill, will test the very best professionals. The religious beliefs and practices of people are far too important to be overlooked.

To conclude this chapter it is necessary to consider a philosophy which centres around man and his place in the universe, that is, without the influence of any deity or supernatural power. Humanism belongs to this way of looking at human life.

Humanism

Humanism emphasizes the importance of man, his nature and place in the universe, and rejects the view that man is a sinful creature who must adjust his way of life to become pure enough to be united with a Supreme Spirit in heaven; with an all-powerful creator of all things. Chaplain Peter Speck (1978) writes:.

> Man as the measure of all things is the keynote in humanistic philosophy, which believes that man can improve his own conditions without supernatural aid, and indeed has a duty to do so. A humanist has faith in man's intellect to bring knowledge and understanding into the world and to solve the moral problems of how to use that knowledge. Respect for one's fellow man, irrespective of class, colour or creed is fundamental together with the moral principles of freedom, tolerance, justice and happiness. The close relationship between mind and body means it is inevitable, says the humanist, that when the body ceases to exist at death the whole life of man is finished. Thus there is no belief in immortality. In the words of Bertrand Russell, 'I believe that when I die I shall rot, and nothing of my ego will survive'.

Humanism is as old as ancient Greece and Rome. However, Humanism as we know it today was founded in an historical movement in Italy during the fourteenth century with the rediscovery of the writings of the classical Greeks and Romans. It used the ancient writings to develop an understanding of human life which was in contrast to the medieval view that man was sinful. The Humanist attitude to the study of human life formed the intellectual essence of the Renaissance. All Humanists agreed that man must be at the centre of their studies and taught that man was a person of dignity and worth and should be respected not despised; in contrast to many medieval scholars who taught that life on earth should be despised because of its evil nature. Humanists rejected the view that man was evil and found widespread acceptance across western Europe. By the sixteenth century, Humanism had spread to France, Germany, the Netherlands and England to become an international fellowship of scholars.

Most authorities agree that much of modern western culture results from

Humanistic achievements, but believe that the great challenge to Humanism is the growing emphasis on science and technology. While accepting that developments in science and technology have increased man's knowledge and power, Humanism has come to represent the growing need for man to use this knowledge and power in a moral way.

Concluding comment

The foregoing does not attempt to give anything like a coverage of the facts relevant to understanding the importance of religious beliefs and practices, and other philosophies, for any ordinary ill person. It only attempts to bring attention to a feature of human life which many of us could overlook in our management of care.

Reference

Speck, P W (1978) Loss and Grief in Medicine, Bailliere Tindall

Further reading

Argyle, M (1958) Religious Behaviour, Routledge
Blackham, H J (1966) Religion in a Modern Society, Constable
Bowker, J (1975) Problems of Suffering in Religions of the World, Cambridge University Press
Brown, D A (1975) A Guide to Religions, S.P.C.K.
Clark, E T (1949) The Small Sects in America, Abingdon Press
Durkheim, E (1954) The Elementary Forms of the Religious Life, translated by J W Swain, Free Press of Glencoe
Herberg, W (1955) Protestant, Catholic, Jew, Doubleday
Lenski, G (1961) The Religious Factor, Doubleday
Neill, S (1958) Anglicanism, Penguin Books
O'Dea, T F (1966) The Sociology of Religion, Prentice Hall
Russell, B (1975) Why I am Not a Christian, Allen and Unwin
Weber, M (1965) The Sociology of Religion, translated by E Fischoff, Methuen
Wilson, B R (1961) Sects and Society, Heinemann
World Book Encyclopedia (1968) Field Enterprises Educational Corporation
Yinger, J M (1957) Religion, Society and the Individual, Macmillan

CHAPTER 3

THE NON-BELIEVER
IN THE HEALTH CARE SITUATION

Introduction

When looking through a nursing card index, in any hospital ward, very rarely does one find the space for the patient's religion filled in as 'none'. When, as a nursing practitioner, I asked the patient his religion and he replied doubtfully, I used to ask if he had been baptized Church of England, and if he agreed I would write that down in the index. Whether I did that to keep my patient records administratively neat, or because I could not accept an ill person not having a religious pigeon-hole, I don't know. Could it have been because I did not seek more insight into the spiritual needs of the patient, to be able to explore with him what he really felt, and to have the courage to write down 'none'? Did I feel competent to support him in his spiritual need without religion?

Increasingly, nurses are meeting patients who do not fit tidily into any religious pigeon-hole. Not only patients, but also doctors, nurses and other health care staff. Doubts may occur at many levels, and be expressed in various ways, and this chapter cannot hope to discuss all possible perspectives. However, it will attempt to explore why certain people can face a serious crisis in their lives, such as a serious illness, without the support of organized religion. Such non-believers come under many labels, e.g. Humanist, neo-Stoic, atheist, or freethinker, but basically they are individuals who do not believe in a life after death along Christian principles, and have reached that decision through intellectual reasoning.

For our purposes, the present chapter employs the term secular — meaning 'worldly' rather than 'sacred' or 'religious' in the accepted sense — to identify the perspective of the non-believer.

It must be accepted that there are many patients who have lapsed in their religious beliefs, and who are unsure. Wilson (1971) claimed that a number of people, when admitted to hospital, will ask to see their local minister, although they haven't practised their religion since childhood. Most of these people are happy to renew their beliefs when faced with hardship and insecurity. They may or may not continue them after the illness has resolved, but that is of no consequence here. Usually, simply asking the patient, 'Would you like to talk to the hospital chaplain, or your local minister?', is sufficient to identify these people. They may need reassurance that the minister or priest will be pleased to talk with them, and will not be rejecting because they seek help under such circumstances.

A more difficult situation for the nurse to cope with is when a family with a deep religious persuasion wish religious sacraments to be performed, while the patient rejects them totally, possibly even in the face of death. This will test the diplomatic skills of the nurse, but both she and the chaplain will know that the patient's expressed wishes are paramount. If the patient continues with this rejection, the nurse will have to support the patient in trying to explain his wishes to his relatives.

To be able to help effectively, the nurse, whatever her own beliefs, should be aware of the possible background to the patient's decision, which might help her to discuss these things with him. After all, non-believers like to discuss religion and philosophy too.

Humanism or non-belief in health and illness

From the time of the Renaissance, there appeared a purely human ideal, rather than the metaphysical ideal of God-like knowledge of Aristotle and Plato. Theological preoccupation was abandoned, and the concentration on the finite, authority and orthodoxy of previous cultures came to be disregarded. This was the beginning of a philosophy, commonly known as Humanism. Humanism, according to Scott (1947) is, 'the effort of men to think, to feel, to act for themselves, and to abide by the logic of results'.

Humanists hope to learn from experience, and the permanent roots of Humanism rest in free enquiry and social agreement. Each individual must decide for himself on the important questions concerning the life he has, and the conduct of it. This means there is no tradition, and no privileged knowledge which is beyond question because it is beyond experience. Rather, there is only experience to be interpreted in the light of further experience, the sole source of all standards of reason and value, forever open to experience (Blackham 1965). Free enquiry is not merely irresponsible thinking, rather it is disciplined thinking, linked with a quest for social agreement.

Humans are social beings, and society is the rules and customs by which conduct is regulated and cooperation ensured and maintained. Society becomes a necessary compromise by which all must abide in order to survive, but the rules of which are always open to review and revision. Different religious beliefs can coincide with such an agreement, e.g. Buddhist, Christian, or Muslim; so one group cannot claim their own belief, built on convention, as the sole grounds for social morality. Social agreement demands tolerance, to avoid claiming the absolute rightness of what one prefers, and to reproach the beliefs of others. Humanists challenge each individual to rely on his own effort and intelligence, even perhaps courage, to become all that he is able, in a world of infinite possibilities. Humanism is, therefore, a guide to the conduct of life, rather than a doctrine of religion, or even philosophy. For the Humanist there is no other life, no existence after death, and no Supreme Being passing judgement.

However, to reject the human longing for reassurance is foolish; rather, this human characteristic tends to run parallel to, rather than replace the longing for intellectual proof. Human beings have, after all, to live by faith in so many aspects of their lives, that to be too analytical — always to demand reason, logic and moral justification — can result in destruction of human relationships. The French philosopher Descartes (1596–1650) claimed that he could maintain complete doubt or scepticism toward any belief or statement that he could not clearly see to be the case. Such a perfect rationality, however, is a denial of human nature, its instincts and the uncertainty of human experience. Consequently, it would be wrong to suggest that a Christian cannot be essentially a Humanist, or that a Humanist must be a complete rationalist, who denies any supernatural explanation for morality. For example, Sir Thomas More, who wrote *Utopia*, was essentially a Humanist, as well as a man of great piety. We all like to delude ourselves that we are rational beings, but our own life events dictate that we are not. Humanism, therefore, when taken out of the abstract, means a deep concern for the development of the total capacities of real people.

The nurse is dealing with real people, in the here and now, which means that, whatever her personal religious belief, she must necessarily be a Humanist. At the same time she can adhere to the religious. The danger is that polarization to either extreme, rational or religious orthodox, will render her incapable of giving nursing care. Admittedly, such extremes are uncommon. Much more common, often more than many nurses are prepared to admit, are oscillations towards one or other end of the continuum. The difficulty of isolating the interface between acceptable or unacceptable rationalistic or religious orthodoxy in nursing is underlined by the subjective nature of the problem. For example, at what point should a nurse teacher, who is perhaps a Humanist, intervene to contrast the expressions of religious orthodoxy of a junior nurse, on the grounds of proselytising? The cue has to come from a third input, usually the patient; but as I mentioned earlier, this can be complicated by the views of close relatives. The most rational approach to seeking a resolution of such a difficult situation may be totally unsuitable, owing to hidden factors such as the personalities of those involved. The nurse teacher may proceed to resolve the problem according to her experience or intuition, but she will probably seek reassurance from others that she has acted in an appropriate manner, whatever her logic dictates, regarding her success or otherwise. Consequently, it would appear that most situations in health care provision imbibe both rational and intuitive, or 'spiritual', components. The objective is to assess and provide the right amounts of both ingredients to an unclear, and often temporary, situation. The ability to achieve this cannot rest solely on rationalistic theory or theological doctrine, and the nurse who has most difficulty, and causes most problems, is the one who cannot be flexible and appropriate within the presenting situation.

The real difficulty lies with those nurses who hold that a revealed religion is a necessity, and act toward the patient accordingly. This is just as unsatisfactory as one who overlooks the need of a patient to reveal his religious beliefs. Consequently, nursing will sustain both the Humanist and the religious, but not extremes of either. The caring situation demands a nurse who can think, and reason out what the situation is. This implies thinking for oneself, and taking responsibility for one's conclusions — it does not mean that one has to be right, or absolutely correct. Real thinking is thinking with a purpose, and with a willingness to correct one's purpose in the light of experience.

Religion in the dock

The main criticism against Humanists is that they are too Utopian in believing that a good environment and a society which keeps human beings happy will make all behave well, knowing it is in their own interests to do so. It is said to be naïve to believe that man is born rational, and to deny the unconscious motive, or the concept of original sin. To Humanists such criticisms are sterile, and one need not deny that people turn to some form of spiritual nourishment when they no longer feel in control of their life events. Because something is irrational is not always sufficient reason for its abolition. Religion, for example, need not be banned when people no longer believe in the myths and dogma traditionally associated with a particular religion.

The need for spiritual nourishment is not only found in individuals who are severely ill in hospital, but also in the whole of mankind, who see the planet drifting toward disaster, whether through a nuclear holocaust, creeping pollution, or over-population. No collective political or social policy is pushing the world in this direction; and no collective policy, from the United Nations or elsewhere, appears to be halting the drift. The Humanist believes it is important to take action, however small, to try to prevent disaster in either the individual or collective situation. Simply abandoning all action, and placing faith in a God of mercy, rather than a God of wrath, is no more a solution than the creation of a scientific 'God' to save the situation. The survival of humanity depends more on understanding the human mind than on being able to prolong human life. Indeed, nurses know that if the will to live is lost, even the most technological of interventions will not succeed. On the other hand, ministers of religion know that promoting the scriptures as sacrosanct canon law, thereby creating anathemas while failing to concentrate on the basic human problems, can be dangerous and weaken morality rather than strengthen it. Morality does not depend solely on a belief in any set of theological doctrines, be they Jewish, Christian, or Muslim. Many criminals, even murderers and terrorists, go to Church on Sunday. The Roman Catholic church, although dominant in Spain and Italy, made no effective resistance to Facism in the 1930s, with all its barbarities. In South Africa, the dominant Protestant churches uphold apartheid, while each year thousands of people lose their lives because of religious conflict. Morality depends chiefly on a social synthesis, and while religion can be supportive of morality it cannot be solely responsible for it.

Humanists claim that to believe something deliberately is meaningless. It is empty to practise religion without having assimilated its teachings, or for no better reason than that the path of reasoning, toward possible agnosticism, is too disruptive to contemplate. Many practise religion for no other reason than that they were taught to do so as children, or because it is expected in their particular society. Many people continue to pray privately, or publically, though few probably believe that a Supernatural Being will meet their individual desires. However, prayer can have the positive effect of concentrating the mind upon purposes which are more likely to be fulfilled if clearly formulated through repetition. Whether by Christian prayer, or Oriental meditation, a concentration of the little understood processes of the human mind may have beneficial effects by indicating a path of action, which might lead to a remedy. Some people find that familiar prayers, or chants, give satisfaction, even though they may no longer believe in the words. People have an unexplained craving for the ceremonial: for example, for the traditional words of the marriage, baptism and burial services. Humanists do not try to find an explanation for such human need, rather they just accept it. Humanists do not simply take the Christian or Jewish world and remove all faith, hope and religion from it. Rather they begin from a standpoint that the natural world contains happiness and pleasure, all of which is perishable but which is to be enjoyed; and the aim is to help others to enjoy it. The use of the mind is cardinal to maintaining an interest in life. The Humanist assumes that life leads to nothing, and that every pretence otherwise is a form of deceit. Consequently, it is important to contribute in any way, however apparently insignificant, up to the moment of death. The end should be the experience itself, rather than the fruits or rewards of experience. Nurses will be aware of patients who 'lived' life to the moment of death; who, despite their pain and disability, actively sought out experience and interaction. They will recall others who began to part themselves from their environment and family long before physical extinction seemed imminent. For the Humanist, death gives the parameters of life, and relationship to human possibilities. Premature death represents an irreplaceable loss.

A human life, therefore, cannot be pigeon-holed and subjected to medical labelling, because it is always open to a wide range of possibilities until the moment of death. Each human life must complete itself, as judged from within, not from without. It is the nurse's role to help the patient, however depressed or disabled he might be, to see what possibilities are open to him. A patient's revealed religion is a support to such endeavours, a source to be utilized, not an end in itself. Whether it springs from secular or religious sources is not relevant; that the patient achieves what he is capable of achieving is, through the development of human self.

The human self, by existing and communicating with others, receives a fresh viewpoint on the world, a form of self-transcendence, through reflecting upon itself and making its own purposes and judgements. Consequently, the self is capable of some self-assessment and transformation. Others act as an *alter ego*, so the face of one's self is reflected back through one's non-self. Therefore, even people professing the same religious beliefs may differ widely in their understanding of it. Indeed, differences occur between one period and another in one life, because of growth and maturity. The reasons for such differences will lie within their experiences, the manner and context in which their religion has been prescribed to them, or the extent to which they can analyse such things. This has led to the wide variety of theological language and symbolism inherent in any religion.

In a situation of change, such as admission to hospital, new influences invite patients to become 'new' people, through experience. They have to find themselves again, to find that commitment which promises to realize their best potential, and therefore to regain their true selves. This is known as existential choice.

We are constantly faced with choices in our everyday lives, but most have no deep significance and we go on living as before. Some choices, however, change our lives; for example, a choice of career in nursing or the ministry, or joining a particular political party. These choices make us decide what kind of life to live, what kind of person to become. Some may believe that there is no choice to be made, because the true self is merely the resolution of the inevitable; an expression of what is already present in us. The self, however, is not at the outset of life all it is to be. Rather it is a dynamic thing which is always growing into what it is to be, and such potential is present from birth. Humanity will remain unfulfilled unless a person has explored, and keeps on exploring, his innermost self and expresses what he finds there, in at least some aspect of his life. However, people differ enormously in the extent to which they have attempted self-exploration. This is important for nurses to remember, because they have to try to assess the degree of insight which a patient has, or appears to need into himself, in his current and future situations. The nurse is helping the patient to explore his potential qualities. As philosopher William James (1902) claimed, 'The divine can mean no single quality, it must mean a group of qualities, by being champions of which in alternation, different men may find different missions'.

The nurse has to be able to recognize and be empathic to a variety of qualities, even though she herself may not have them; after all, to recognize the causes of alcoholism is not to be an alcoholic. This recognition will take place whether or not the patient has a revealed religion. When we talk about religion, we are dealing with abstract, cosmic symbolism; but when we talk about a patient's religion, we are dealing with a private and personal phenomena, with realities, because the subjective cannot be omitted or suppressed.

However, Humanists believe that such personalization can have a deleterious effect at times, in that Christians frequently restrict the scope of ethics into a narrow class of 'personal' sins. Not only does this increase the individual sense of guilt, but the individual can be averted from the many social injustices in their local community. For example, a Victorian patriarchy might have condemned an individual for adultery, yet employed children in factories at slave wages. Even today, being dishonest to a friend might be condemned vigorously, yet failing to speak out against racism or sectarianism is not. A different example might be how the elderly in our community are inundated with parties and food baskets at Christmas, but ignored and neglected for the rest of the year. Martin Luther once said that, if one preaches the Gospel in all aspects with the exception of the issues which deal specifically with one's time, one is not preaching the Gospel at all.

The Humanist wants to change the structures of society which cause unnecessary casualties, rather than attempting merely to retrieve the remains of such casualties. He seeks communities of caring defiance against the evils of society, and may claim that churches are largely comfortable clubs of conformity. Such conformity rests on the complicated social interactions with significant others, in which one develops and maintains one's personal view of reality, and which supports the validity of certain ideas. If such supporting structures are no longer available, doubt, anxiety and insecurity may arise. Therefore, it is easier for a practising religionist to feel secure in his particular 'truth' than the non-believer, for his community provides therapy against a creeping doubt. Human beings need to feel a sense of belonging to a community, which has resulted in the vast array of religious and quasi-religious sects that have sprung up in the twentieth century. Each one is seeking support against his own individual doubt. The determination with which some people cling to their beliefs, therefore, is not necessarily a function of the rationality of the grounds on which they hold them. A patient may not have any desire to explore his religious beliefs with either minister or nurse, and may settle happily for what he has, perhaps fearing loss and insecurity.

It is often said that faith, or lack of faith, means the possession of logical certitude. However, both believer and non-believer can be equally subject to doubt. Faith means a commitment to a transformation which is open ended, that even when the early stages are complete the end cannot as yet be conceptualized. So the religionist accepts not just the doctrine, but a way of life and doctrine as being one and the same. The non-believer, including the Humanist, claims to be able to live the system of life without doctrine, by using a store of knowledge and his perception of reality. Our perception constitutes our reality, and we cannot devise any alternative; and without reality we cannot function, or survive. Our reality is that our human morality is something less than perfect, something less than God-like, and consequently we live by laws and regulations and are motivated to behave ourselves by the ultimate sanction of punishment. The religionist might claim that we live in a state of love and trust with God; but cannot this be said to be an act of emotional dependence, akin to a child's love and trust of a parent who nevertheless abuses him? Does not such dependence inhibit our growth as independent individuals, when carried to extremes of passivity? Whether a patient sees his God as a God of wrath, demanding confession, or a God of love, demanding worship, the non-believer claims that this can divert and inhibit the humanity of the patient, at a time when he needs to think as clearly and as rigorously as his abilities will allow. To indulge in the proposition of the intentionality of God, at a time of crisis, can result in a fatalism which weakens the critical consciousness at a time when the patient needs it most.

No absolute security is possible. The anxiety of death and helplessness in the face of fate produces a quest for security, which is perfectly normal, and doesn't have to be 'cured'. What has to be treated is the misplaced or unrealistic anxiety about illness and possible death to a point where it affects the person, in that they are self-limiting in their existence. Progress is achieved when óne begins to accept the fact that even if all external things are right, real happiness would still depend on one's own character, and being able to live with its flaws. It is easier to claim to know the flaws in others than in oneself. Self-exploration, to the Humanist, is not the same as the self-contempt or self-love that is sometimes evident in the religious.

The nurse may find herself disappointed at her own behaviour or thoughts in certain nursing situations. She has not lived up to her own ideal of what she should be. Such disappointment may lead her to seek a form of revenge, first upon self, and then upon others. Such egotism can sometimes be seen in a nurse who claims not to spare herself; and who by implication has the right not to spare others the same inconvenience. For example, the ward sister who as a learner had to cope with a busy surgical ward at night may say brusquely to a learner, 'I did it, so why can't you?' Such a sister may be denying the anguish and ineptitude she had endured, unconsciously saying, 'I found out that I was only human, and couldn't do everything, now it's your turn'.

It is superficially easy for the nurse to give explanations to patients about disability, embarrassment, pain and dying. However, most nurses are young men and women, most of whom have never actually experienced the conditions or situations they are attempting to explain away. Why is it that the elderly ward cleaner, uninhibited by the constraint of professional infallibility, can be such a source of comfort to many patients? Simply because she has the humility of life experience to *share* with the patients. She has, perhaps, witnessed the death of several family members, endured childbirth, operations, and being stripped naked in front of a large group of medical students. She is a comfort because she can share where the majority of nurses cannot, or do not appear to be able to find the time. On one psychiatric ward I worked on, the white, middle-class neurotic patients received their medication from the nurse, their psychoanalysis from the psychiatrist, but their comfort and life direction from a large, coloured and illiterate cleaning lady, whose contented, earthy and outspoken life philosophy filled a yearning for security which no professional appeared to offer. If a young nurse has not had the experience of the patient, she must try to let the patient share it with her, and through her, rather than offer explanations to the patient based on physiological or theological doctrine. Through such humility, the nurse will grow with experience.

It is easier to maintain a philosophical calm toward one's own misfortune, than those of one's loved ones. A mother might endure her own pain with equanimity, but be devastated and helpless in respect of pain in her child. However, even in the face of the greatest misfortune, one must not become shut up in a world of sorrow, for a life dominated by a single passion is incapable of any kind of wisdom. Believers might say that it is better to see misfortune in relation to causes, and as part of the whole order of nature; that these are only misfortunes to the individual, not to the universal nature of an ultimate harmony. For many, it is comforting to reflect that human life with all its suffering is an infinitesimal part of the life of the Universe. A non-believer is unlikely to accept this. Particular events are what they are, and do not become different when absorbed into the whole; nothing that happens later can make an act good that was bad. Television, and other media, bring scenes of inhumanity and death into our homes. For the first time in history, we can see a child in Africa actually die from starvation, while in the comfort of our armchair. In the same programmes we see the political leaders of those countries, surrounded by a military, bristling with weaponry, shouting political ideology at each other. Also, for the first time in history, man rather than divine judgement can destroy all civilization, by the use of nuclear weapons. It becomes increasingly difficult, when under constant bombardment of human, and often self-inflicted misery, to see suffering in terms of any Universal plan, even within the purview of free will.

Philosophers such as Leibniz (1646–1716) attempted to explain this by claiming that God's actions have the same end of freedom or free will. He claimed that God always acts for the best, but is under no logical compulsion to do so. Another philosopher, Thomas Aquinas (1226–74) claimed that God cannot act contrary to the laws of logic, but as God can decree whatever is logically possible, it leaves God a great latitude of choice. Modern theologians have tried to explain free will as due to God's limited power, that He is not omnipotent or omnipresent, but is more wise and powerful than us.

Non-believers do not try to explain suffering this way, because they have rejected all three conflicting faces of a metaphysical Being — namely the God of Power of the Old Testament, the God of Love of the New Testament and the intellectual God of the modern-day theologians. Indeed, some modern Protestant religions have rejected the God of the reformers, such as Calvin, and have reverted to the Old Testament concept of the God of Punishment and Wrath. The non-believer therefore, is not satisfied with any 'proof' that a God exists, in any dimension. Such arguments that a Supreme Being is present in the Universe appear to centre on the idea that a Being who possesses all perfections is better if He exists than if He does not. From which it follows that, if He does not exist, He cannot be the best possible Being. For today's society, past arguments do not seem very convincing, but non-believers have to admit that it is easier to feel doubt than to point out precisely where the fallacy lies.

The concept of heaven, or life after death, rests on the presence or absence of a 'soul', which in turn rests on there being a concept of 'self'. Philosopher David Hume (1711–76) repudiated the concept of self. He claimed that one cannot enter intimately into 'myself'. One cannot catch oneself at any time without a perception, and can never observe anything but that perception. Therefore, one does not know whether self exists, except as a bundle of perceptions, e.g. happy or sad, loving or hating. Consequently, the concept of self cannot enter into any part of our knowledge, and abolishes all supposed knowledge of the 'soul', and pushes us back into probabilities. According to Hume, we must believe we have a self, and we must believe we have a soul, as we cannot experience either. However, even if the soul exists, the non-believer might claim that there is no evidence to show the purpose or objective of its existence. The concept of 'soul' cannot survive outside of a religious philosophy.

The Humanist suggests that man is a sensitive being, capable of reasoning, and of acquiring moral ideals, and this leads to the non-believer giving a high value to education. Education, in its widest sense, is important if man is to attempt to actualize all his potentialities. Humanists believe that such potentialities are inexhaustible, because the creativity of nature breaks into the consciousness of man. As they actualize, potentialities then release further potential in turn, whether in the horizontal, vertical, futuristic or temporal. Consequently, Humanism sets out to transform reality to the demands of reason. It relieves the anxiety of meaninglessness by activity, and the threat of guilt by accepting the shortcomings and mistakes both of individuals and of societies as unavoidable, while believing in improvement through education and the releasing of creative possibilities. This is the core of the nursing experience.

The non-believer attempts to accept doubt, a process common to all. Happold (1966) described the doubt process as follows:

> As souls, accustomed to rely on the dogmatism, doctrinal and historical elements of religion, become more spiritually mature, the particular symbolic structure of their religion tends to collapse, the image of God to which they have been accustomed fades, the familiar props and landmarks are left behind. As a result they feel a sense of emptiness, aridity and desolation.

For those to whom, in the past, religion was little more than a form of escapism, or a conformity to a social requirement, doubt may simply cause the individual to seek refuge in materialism. For the more introspective, doubt can be more painful, faith may be lost and life begins to have no meaning. Alternatively, doubt can lead to more spiritual maturity, perhaps more religious, perhaps more secular. It is probably sterile to attempt to define a correct spiritual maturity, for as the prophet Krishna claimed, there are two ways to reach the highest good: for the contemplative, the path of spiritual knowledge; and for the active the path of dedicated action. In the Bible, in the story of Martha and Mary, Christ emphasized the importance of the contemplative but did not, as is sometimes interpreted, denigrate action as a form of worship. An interesting anecdote concerns a young novice monk who asked his spiritual adviser for spiritual instruction. 'Have you had breakfast yet?' asked the Master, 'Yes', answered the novice. 'Well then, go wash the dishes', came the reply. A nurse who finds herself capable of 'washing the dishes' for a patient will always find herself capable of developing spiritual maturity regardless of her religion.

Anxiety, fear and self-affirmation

According to Tillich (1969), anxiety is reduced by producing and preserving certitude, examples of which might include religious sacraments, or belief in the physician's expertise. The patient needs to gain a balance between courage and fear. In addition, he needs to adjust to being a part of the health care situation, but the role he is normally expected to play is a passive one. He has become separated from the balance he had achieved between his selfishness as an individual, and his participation in his group. He now finds that participation in a new group is demanded, to the detriment of his individuality. The affirmation of his self-concept has been damaged, and his efforts to re-establish himself may be undermined by the attitudes of health carers. When faced with the possibility of death, and the annihilation of the physical self, the pressure to give in to total participation is increased, to become totally passive, to follow medical and nursing orders, and to withdraw from decision making regarding self.

Another form of withdrawal regarding self is present in life. For example, in some Eastern and Communist countries which have resorted to nationalism rather than reasoned socialism, self is not expressed in individual terms but in respect of the group, whether the family, place of employment, or Party. To strive for individualism is regarded as antisocial, to be corrected by the whole community; and in act of contrition, the 'sinner' stands before his group and regains acceptance through confession. In the religious, however, the main threat to the individual is one of non-being, when the contrite sinner stands alone before his God. He is anxious because no one else can stand with him, but the Christian church attempts to relieve this anxiety by its collective traditions, sacraments and authority — a collective preparation to give courage to stand alone.

The non-believer has already made a conscious decision to stand alone or to stand apart, and consciously to rejoin the group from will, because he has realized the benefits of social cooperation. He does not suffer a fear of being alone, or the fear of the loneliness of a metaphysical retribution. However, he differs from the Communist in that he refuses to relinquish his own self-being to the collective; rather he sees himself worthy of self-identity and fulfilment. He shares with the Communist, however, something of the feeling of the eternal in the continuing existence of the essence of mankind, as opposed to individual immortality.

From the moment we are born we are dying, so the moment of death is simply the completion of the dying process. Few people fear death; they fear the minutes or hours before death. Happiness, by contrast, is the ability to feel a sudden release of joy at having controlled fear or anxiety, of inhibiting our baser desires, and simply being. The patient has a desire to feel the happiness of being well, he fears dying or deformity, and has to restore his sense of wholeness in the face of hardship. He has to learn to control anxiety or even to relinquish it, through the acceptance of being what he is, and the affirmation of himself as an individual. His ability to achieve this will depend, in part, on how he is accepted by others, particularly nurses. If the nurse tries to understand, and accept his pain, his deformity, or his death, and tries to be empathic to the experience which the patient is enduring, the patient can give of himself as a human being, up to the second of his death. By having the courage to share, and thereby having the courage to live, the patient may have the courage to die. Hope and fear are emotions which depend on viewing the future as uncertain, but the non-believer is unlikely to view the future this way, because for him there is no future after death. Suffering, therefore, is not allowed to conquer his being. The nurse can only help if she feels confident in her own self-identity, whether or not this is supported by her own religious beliefs.

Self-affirmation and self-preservation are synonymous in that both imply the overcoming of something which potentially threatens or denies the self (Tillich 1969). According to the philosopher Nietzche (1844–1900), the will that commands itself is the creative will, the will that strives to become. In contrast, the submissive self seeks to escape the pain of hurting and of being hurt. Even in physical illness, the will to strive and overcome is not entirely lost. In mental illness, however, where self-negation is evident, the will to strive is rarely manifest. In such psychotic illnesses as schizophrenia, the detachment from reality might be described as a loss of the will to 'live' while lacking the courage to die. Therefore, the patient exists in a state of limbo, unable to become what others expect of him and unable to strive for self-identity. He cannot explore, accept and grow within and from his hardship; he is succumbing to anxiety and guilt. Although psychotropic drugs will help to break down the barriers to communication which the patient has erected, they will not help him to develop a self-identity which will enable him to contain his anxieties. Such a building up of his self-being must come about with the help of other human beings.

Tillich (1969) claimed that anxiety is the existential awareness of non-being. 'It is not', he claims, 'the abstract knowledge or non-being which produces anxiety, but the awareness that non-being is a part of one's being'. The non-believer has come to terms, perhaps better than most, with the anxiety of non-being, of knowing that he has to die, and that is the end. Fear, as opposed to anxiety, is a definite object which can be faced, analysed, endured and overcome. Fear is being afraid of something, e.g. of dying. What brings about anxiety is not the act of dying, but the possible negativity associated with the implications of death. We fear the act of dying, its possible pain etc., but we are anxious about its objective, that is the after-death of non-being. Philosophers such as Spinoza (1632–77) sought to establish an outlook which could liberate men from the oppression of fear. He wrote, 'A free man thinks of nothing less than of death, and his wisdom is a meditation, not of death, but of life'. By accepting the concept that there is no life after death, that it means oblivion as beings, the non-believer reduces his anxiety, although he will fear the act of dying, as will all human beings. It is here that the nurse can help the patient — to meet death with minimal discomfort and dignity, and by letting him exist in his individuality right up to the moment of death, e.g. by using drugs to control pain, or psychosis, but not to stupefy. To deny the patient this is to emphasize the objectlessness of his being.

Patients do not fear the act of being stripped naked in front of others, but they are anxious about its impact on their being, the dignity of their individual adultness, the hurt of not being in control of the situation. Human beings seek therefore, to turn their anxiety into fear, through identifying objects of fear, no matter what, so it can be faced and overcome. One can only talk about non-being in terms of being, as one defines unconsciousness only in terms of consciousness, as non-being and unconsciousness have no qualities. Consequently, the patient expresses his fear of the imminent operation, the helplessness under the anaesthetic, and the concern of what will be the 'new' him after the surgery.

As long as the nurse can isolate such objects of fear, anxiety can be overcome. Anxiety cannot be tackled directly, because it has no object, in that it negates every object. The patient expresses helplessness, which expresses itself in a loss of direction, inadequate reactions, and a lack of intention or will. The source of this threat is non-being, which lacks any objectivity on which the patient can focus, explore and overcome. It is not helpful simply to state that anxiety is fear of the unknown, for as unknown, by its very nature, it cannot be known. The nurse must help the patient to focus on an object of his fear, e.g. anaesthetic, and to allay fear through providing adequate information. She cannot help the anxiety of non-being, she can only hope to reduce it, or re-shape it into something more objective, a fear, which the nurse and patient can tackle together. She can never hope to overcome anxiety in herself, or the patient, for non-being is present even when an immediate threat, e.g. death, is absent. As Tillich (1969) pointed out, 'It stands behind the insecurity and loneliness of our social and individual experience'.

While the religious overcome such anxiety through belief in life after death, that the being continues to exist through the soul, the non-believer relieves anxiety through acts of self- and social affirmation, through a collective eternalism, rather than through a Christian individual salvation. The nurse increases her own spiritual and self-affirmation through discovering not only the fear object of the patient, but also the fear object in herself. However, spiritual affirmation cannot be intentionally produced, as an avoidance in the nurse, of the anxiety of the meaninglessness of life. Daily, she witnesses the apparent purposelessness of suffering and death. She might try every explanation but nothing might explain satisfactorily, and indeed might produce a deeper anxiety concerning the meaninglessness of it all. She may then resort to erecting barriers to suffering, and become remote from the patients, steeped in professionalism. Patients sometimes call such nurses 'hard', because they have become separated from rather than participating in the illness experience of the patients. It is only in such sharing that she will find her own self, and her spiritual identity — it cannot be taught, forced or manufactured, and it will be unique to her.

That is why the nurse can give and share with patients irrespective of her own religion, or lack of it, because the experiences she has feed her own wisdom. She can only take by giving, and she can only give what the patient needs if she is prepared to take from him in return. The technological environment of modern hospital care reduces such sharing, to the detriment of the nurse's self-affirmation, as well as the patient's. The machine helps us to avoid asking questions, or seeking answers. It gives us a result on which to take action. While a vital instrument in the physical well-being of the patient, if it becomes the sole focus of our care reaction it diverts us from asking other, perhaps equally important questions, such as, 'What does the *patient* want to become?', and 'How can I help him become?', rather than, 'How do I reduce his serum potassium level?'. The restoration of electrolyte balance may be necessary to save the patient's life, but the 'self' of both patient and nurse might be being sacrificed. It is a question of balance. This is so whether or not the patient or nurse have a revealed religion. Religion is an adjunct and support to the essence of self-affirmation, provided it is not used as a prop, or as another form of chemotherapy. The wise priest or minister recognizes this and can even help the non-believer through discussion and exploration of experience. Some ministers of religion refuse to speak to patients of other, or of no religion. They are using their own doctrine as a barrier to their own experience, to developing their own identity. Such ministers are denying themselves far more than they are seeking to protect, namely the sharing of the opportunity to grow in wisdom and maturity. The greatest waste lies in the denial of self and of the potential of self. Authoress Katherine Mansfield wrote, when near death, 'I want to be all that I am capable of becoming' — this is the very essence of the nursing experience.

References

Blackham, H J (Editor) (1965) Objections to Humanism, Constable

Happold, F C (1966) Religious Faith and Twentieth Century Man, Darton, Longman and Todd

James, W (1902) The Varieties of Religious Experience: A Study of Human Nature, The Modern Library

Scott, G (1947) The Architecture of Humanism, Constable

Tillich, P (1969) The Courage to Be, Collins

Wilson, M (1971) The Hospital, A Place of Truth? — A Study of the Role of the Hospital Chaplain, University of Birmingham, Institute for the Study of Worship and Religious Architecture

CHAPTER 4

SUFFERING THROUGH ILLNESS

What is suffering?

Suffering is described as a condition of being in pain; a state of distress, agony or misery. Hunger causes suffering. Torture causes suffering. The poet Longfellow wrote, 'Know how sublime a thing it is to suffer and be strong'. Sismondi believed that, 'Suffering is the surest means of making us truthful to ourselves'. But what is suffering? Subhadra Bhikshu tells us that, 'To be born is to suffer; to grow old is to suffer; to die is to suffer; to lose what is loved is to suffer; to be tied to what is not loved is to suffer; to endure what is distasteful is to suffer. In short, all the results of individuality, of separate self-hood, necessarily involve suffering.' Father Francis McNutt (1977) wrote, 'Suffering is a part of life ... some of that suffering is caused by sickness, to help us to do something that will make us well. Of its very nature it occupies centre stage in our attention, until we move to change. It is the body crying out for help, for pity.'

Hitherto, we have given a condition or state the title 'suffering', and the person, the object of the condition, is called the 'sufferer'. We are familiar with notions of suffering through the disciplines of psychology, biology, philosophy, history and religion, but even with personal experience we can only describe suffering from the outside; as if it were strange and unreal. The great number of stories of personal experiences of sorrow and affliction lead us to believe that suffering is a reality which has continued throughout the history of mankind. Suffering is real and belongs to all of us. I do not want to overdo this line of argument because the same can be used for 'hating', or 'loving' but, because it is relevant to care giving, I am reluctant to leave suffering as just a notion of something that happens to people who become ill and might die. For example, merely to say to a patient, 'I know how you feel', and to leave it at that, is to use so many empty words just for the sake of saying them.

The need for intervention

It is not possible to adopt any other person's perceptions and reactions in any meaningful way; especially when the person may not have full measure of his own thoughts and feelings about the matter under discussion. To venture that we know how people feel, or might feel, about their suffering requires insights not merely into pain, but of a general kind into problems of dependency, loss of self-esteem, guilt, loss of pleasure, or loss of relationships with family and friends. Even if the sufferer does tell us about his affliction, and allows an exhaustive clinical examination, we are only gaining indications of his suffering; ambiguous signals which may lead to a great deal of misunderstanding of the complete state of the person's dilemma. It may be that the sufferer does not know the truth of his suffering. The difficulty takes shape from the way the various factors of the state of suffering affect each other. None of the contributory factors, e.g. pain, fear, loss of independence etc., has much meaning in isolation. Isolation of any single factor is arbitrary. Suffering exists through the interrelationship of its various factors. General feelings of uncertainty, powerlessness and frustration become unavoidable if one factor becomes all important. Despite this, health care professionals continue to give the impression that the patient's total suffering belongs to his pathology. It is necessary to think beyond mere tissue explanations of suffering, and to allow ourselves and our patients a broader perspective; we don't have any right to do otherwise.

Several authors argue that patients pick up the concern of care givers about the effectiveness of treatment, but are not likely to receive much support in dealing with other future concerns. Such authors claim that care givers try to maintain the patient's optimism, encouraging him to avoid thinking about death while, at the same time, failing to deal with his feelings of uncertainty and frustration. For example, Castles and Murray (1979) claimed that:

> When the patient has no opportunity to handle his feelings, he is denied a chance fully to understand his problems, to integrate the concept of his

vulnerability into his self-concept, and to work through the meaning or sense of his suffering. Help with this derivation of meaning is likely to come from religion or from a significant family member, rather than be part of the medical therapeutic effort.

While accepting that suffering is personal, and outside of the consciousness of other individuals, sufferers may seek a more complete understanding of their suffering from these others. Help can be offered through adopting both an objective and shared view of the patient's suffering by asking, 'In what sense is any sufferer the subject of his suffering?'. He is of course subject in the sense of being personally involved, but whether he becomes subject to the experience by lying down before its influence and thereby adding to his suffering or by accepting suffering in a positive way are outcomes which can be influenced by the interventions of nurses, clerics, and family members. How one copes with personal suffering, or the suffering of others, is influenced by such things as one's state of health, the quality of care, and religion.

The person in health

Most healthy people think, occasionally, about suffering through illness. A few may try to think what it would be like to die through suffering. However, for obvious reasons, well people will find these imagined roles difficult to assume. Their thinking may have been triggered by a headache or unexplained pain, but most people believe that their infrequent headaches or vague pains are merely annoyances; undesirable and frustrating, but not things of significance. Talcott Parsons (1951) claimed that

> Most people have an unrealistic bias in the direction of confidence that 'everything will be all right', that is, they are motivated to underestimate the chances of their falling ill, especially seriously ill (the minority of hypochondriacs is the obverse), and if they do they tend to overestimate the chances of a quick recovery.... One possible reaction is to attempt to deny illness or various aspects of it, to refuse to 'give in' to it.

There is reason to believe that most healthy individuals view suffering as a general fate to be experienced soon enough.

In this connection, some patients undoubtedly appreciate the opportunity to accept their illness, whereas for others the opportunity to 'deny' may be appropriate and acceptable. Also, any ordinary person who has formed close relationships and lives a normal lifestyle will undoubtedly be exposed to the sufferings of relatives and others and will experience deep sorrow from time to time. But the tendency is to try to 'get on with living' as nearly in the usual pattern as possible, to avoid too much concern with the prospect of suffering or its implications, and to return to thought and feeling for the normal happenings of everyday existence. While the healthy person must think at times, however briefly and intermittently, about the sufferings of others, his interest priorities will normally exclude thoughts of personal suffering.

The interest priorities of the healthy person belong to those elements of his cultural pattern of life, namely his social world with family, friends and acquaintances, which may serve as means or ends for his use and enjoyment, and which are within his actual or potential grasp. His priorities fit, in a general way, into an incoherent system. His tactics belong to a short-term strategy with his plans for different aspects of life, and various social roles, deviating with situational change. The thinking patterns of the ordinary person derive from a blueprint, or ready-made scheme of reference, for almost any situation which normally occurs in his social life. Schutz (1971) wrote, 'The world seems to him at any given moment as stratified in different levels of relevance, each of them requiring a different degree of knowledge'. Yet, socialized man is incapable of becoming acquainted with all relevancies with equal thoroughness, regardless of their degree of significance. The ready-made, standardized scheme of reference is inadequate under special conditions, e.g. suffering, in the cultural and social systems. The attitude of the healthy individual with respect to suffering is incoherent and lacking in reflection. 'I would rather drop dead than lie suffering' is the kind of response offered by well people and, for many, there is no alternative response.

The new sufferer

McGilloway (1979) claimed that:

> Socialized man does not normally quest for certainty under normal or everyday circumstances. He tends to accept the ready-made pattern of living handed down to him as a guide, in all the situations which normally occur within the concrete social world. All he wants is information of likelihood and insight into the chances or risks the situation potentiates.

The well person is able to speak calmly about suffering through illness, that is until it seizes upon his own personal life.

For the new sufferer a crisis arises; especially for the person who is admitted to hospital, where the culture pattern reveals that the applicabilty of the ready-made is now confined to a specific historical situation. McGilloway and Donnelly (1977) argued that it is only when he is confronted with breaking points in the socially structured round of daily behaviour that any socialized man is importantly and seriously challenged. They claim that:

> The ill person in hospital lives in conditions of uncertainty; events of crucial significance for his wellbeing are beyond his prevision. The combination of helplessness, technical incompetence and emotional and social stress, described by McGilloway (1976), which define him as a patient, is complicated by the ever-present characteristic 'contingency', which refers to the fact that all human ventures, no matter how carefully planned or expertly executed, are liable to disappointment. The person, whether by a self-motivated process or the motivations of relatives or diagnostic agencies, finds himself in a defined framework, which is different, in which he is institutionally defined as a patient and his need institutionally categorized. For him the definition of reality is difficult; important aspects of self-understanding and self-identification are disturbed, and his future prospects are uncertain.

The patient, a well person until a few hours ago, who could speak calmly about suffering through illness, now discovers that the management of problems which fall within the scope of his suffering cannot be taken for granted. The new sufferer becomes a person who has to place in question nearly everything that seemed to be unquestionable just a few hours earlier. The system of knowledge of suffering, incoherent and only partially questioned, if at all, but generally adequate within the concrete world of the healthy, is no longer sufficiently coherent and clear to give him a reasonable chance of understanding relevant phenomena within the world of suffering. McGilloway (1979) stated that:

> It is seen that, for the new patient, the reality of the standardized socialization scheme becomes unworkable when former experiences fail to suffice for further situations; when former solutions fail to meet problems and the knowledge handed down by significant others ceases to be reliable; when it is not enough to know 'just something' about dealing with problems in order to manage and control them.

It was implied earlier that suffering comprises an interrelationship of factors, and that the range of possible complexities in this sphere is very great. The factors are, however, structured by the nature and degree of illness — circumstances and consequences — in certain relatively definite ways. In this connection, Parsons (1951) wrote:

> Perhaps the most definite point is that for the 'normal' person illness … constitutes a frustration of expectancies of his normal life pattern. He is cut off from his normal spheres of activity, and many normal enjoyments. He is often humiliated by his incapacity to function normally. His social relationships are disrupted to a greater or lesser degree. He may have to bear discomfort or pain, which is hard to bear, and he may have to face serious alterations of his prospects for the future, in the extreme but by no means uncommon case, the termination of his life.

How health care professionals react, through their therapeutic efforts, to the separate factors of suffering will inevitably influence the nature of the relationships of these factors. Moreover, whether ill people pay explicit attention to it or not, what care givers do, and the way they do it, inevitably influences the emotional state of their patients and this will often have an important influence on the state of their suffering.

Many theologians and lay people accept that the purpose of pain and the suffering it causes can be beneficial in physical and redemptional ways. (Redemptive suffering will be discussed in a later section.) They put forward the argument that pain, and other symptoms, draw the sufferer's attention to some malfunction and, if prolonged or severe, the sufferer is likely to attend to the problem. McNutt (1977) wrote, 'When I'm sick, the pain concentrates my attention on my body or emotions until I do something to get rid of the sickness….' Given this kind and level of argument, perhaps a few words may be helpful about the relation of symptoms to important illnesses and the impact they might have on the attitudes of ordinary people.

Certain conditions, for example pyelonephritis, a common illness in women, present with symptoms that may disappear within a few days, even without treatment, and yet the disease continues to destroy tissue. Symptoms of nausea, loss of weight, anorexia, and changes of bowel habit may be manifestations of a cancer of the colon, but such symptoms are so common, in separateness, that ordinary people will tend to ignore them. There are innumerable everyday discomforts and physical irregularities that come and go which, while most people ignore them, could belong to serious conditions. We grow into adulthood with a history of aches, gastric upsets, tiredness, constipation, or diarrhoea. Many false alarms are raised, or unnecessary heed paid to some of these discomforts. Indeed, it would be unrealistic to attend a physician on every occasion one experiences a pain or suffers a minor illness. We only concentrate our attentions on 'sickness' when it interferes with the necessary activities of our lives. In general, without professional advice, we are not qualified to recognize the significance of symptoms or to choose between them.

When the body does emit warnings most of these signals are ambiguous, and many people refuse to accept them as important. Attitudes to health vary among people. Some attempt to adapt to their symptoms and refuse to accept the status of sufferer; for instance, they accept an arthritic pain as natural to ageing, or breathlessness as resulting from too many cigarettes. Others will assume a role that requests help, perhaps more help than some professionals see as necessary or feasible. Another reaction is to deny that a problem exists. An extreme example of denial is the knowledgeable woman who is aware of a lump in her breast and does nothing about it for fear of embarrassment, loss of dignity, or hearing the truth. Perplexing and irrational as this woman's behaviour may be, her fears will be very real and her mental as well as physical suffering will be extreme as the disease progresses.

Fortunately, such instances are atypical. The normal reaction is to seek help optimistically. Those who have ignored symptoms are apt to present with reactions of shock and anxiety, when an illness develops, especially if the condition is diagnosed as chronic because of the state of irreversible impairment.

The person suffering critical illness

For a large proportion of new sufferers the health care team appear to have a straightforward task, their knowledge and skill allowing adequate ways and means for accomplishing recovery and cure. There is, of course, the matter of dealing with the emotional and social reactions of ill people and their relatives. However, when the prognosis is good it is usually only necessary to work competently to ensure a cure for the patient. Despite such competence, the critically ill person may suffer intense pain and experience a sense of helplessness and possible bewilderment, resulting in difficult problems of physical, emotional and social adjustment. The sufferer, not knowing what is happening, can only take his cues from others. He may have recovered consciousness while being carried in an ambulance, on a stretcher, or hospital trolley. He might find himself in the bed of an intensive care unit without any recollection as to the cause of his being there. He might have suffered some form of confusion for hours, and now feels excruciating pain, stupefaction and fear. Alternatively, he may have to adjust to the idea of a change in his body image whether from internal changes, for example in heart disease, or because of external disfigurement as in facial burns. In the meanwhile, his pain, bewilderment and various fears, in the hushed urgency of the critical care unit, will be sufficient to cause him suffering.

Burrell and Burrell (1977) claimed that the management of the care of the critically ill patient might cause him to suffer additional stress. Their description of the atmosphere of the intensive care unit, of 'hushed urgency', allows us to visualize a person in bed, through injury or illness, partially immobilized by intravenous tubing, electrodes and catheters. He may even have restraints on his extremities to keep the various tubes in place, and his ability to speak may be inhibited or removed because of a tracheostomy tube. He can't feed himself, take a drink of water, or do any of those things commensurate with adult integrity. He will suffer sleeplessness, interruptions of sleep from pain and repeated examinations, observations of vital signs and a variety of treatments such as injections. An overhead light may be shining continuously. He will be exposed to the groans, coughing or delirious statements of other critically ill patients. Other noises will include the sounds of respirators, monitors and suction machines, or voices giving technical directions about himself or other patients. He will probably hear, either vaguely or clearly, discussions of his own or other patient conditions. His sense of time will be upset by illness or the effect of medications and, when they are allowed to visit, the worried expressions upon the faces of his loved ones may add to his plight.

Consequently, it is important to remember that the dilemma of any person in the situation of sufferer belongs not only to the illness state, but also to such feelings of helplessness, uncertainty and frustration — increased by a lack of relevant knowledge — and to problems of physical, emotional and social adjustment.

The person suffering chronic illness

The person with a chronic illness, who will require long-term care, must assimilate the prognosis into his way of life. Life is prolonged but it is different from life before the diagnosis of his illness. Many long-term patients, including those suffering heart dysfunction, cancer, or renal disease, may have to live with uncertainty about life and death. They could have received treatments, and experienced remissions, yet they must persist with more and more treatments. While they may be well improved, but not curable, they must live under sentence of death for an unpredictable number of years. Many chronic illnesses are not dramatic, for example bronchitis and arthritis; however, all persons suffering chronic illness can experience important incapacities which necessitate role changes and alter relationships with family and friends. Sometimes their illness may even require termination of wage earning, with reliance on State welfare.

The life of the person suffering chronic illness is centred on his disease or disorder. Time is structured around the management of his illness, with short periods in hospital, frequent visits to the general practitioner, and continuous monitoring of his condition. Gabriel (1981) described the typical lifestyle of a person who receives haemodialysis treatment for chronic renal disease:

> At first, the patient may need only a weekly dialysis, but within a few months it becomes necessary to dialyse twice weekly to maintain health. For a person working full time, or a housewife with a family, dialysis is usually performed from the evening to the early hours of the next morning. This is restrictive on the social life of the family. In addition, normal family holidays are not possible as most dialysis equipment is insufficiently portable. From the friction developed between the healthy and the less healthy spouse, marital discord and divorce are not uncommon.

Castles and Murray (1979) claimed that, 'These patients are experienced interpreters of symptoms in relation to favorable and unfavorable progress. They tend to live from day to day, often with feelings of mild depression and loss of control, holding onto time and bidding for more of it, always considering the probability of a new drug or treatment'.

The pattern of living of the person with a chronic illness presents the patient and those close to him with problems of emotional and social adjustments. For any normal person, disablement, helplessness and the risk of death constitute basic disturbances of the expectations by which he lives; disturbances which cannot be emotionally accepted without the accompaniments of strain and, hence, without difficult adjustments for both patient and family. Relief may come from religion, and this will be discussed later. The following passage from Castles and Murray (1979) allows further consideration of the possible kinds of social adjustment made by the patient on behalf of family and friends. They claimed that:

> A gradual social withdrawal occurs, particularly for those persons with a diagnosis of cancer, for former friends frequently express fear of catching the disease, or fail to offer needed support. Friends expect the patient to look death-like, to be in constant pain or to be unable to perform ordinary tasks or enjoy ordinary pleasures. These patients, therefore, are likely to conceal evidence of the disease from others in order to avoid their withdrawal or rejection.

The remarkable advances of the last 30 years in the field of health care have given significant hope of extended life to many people. Consequently, it must be expected that more people will survive critical illness to become long-term sufferers; for others suffering will end in death.

Suffering through dying

It is impossible that anything so natural, so necessary and so universal as death, should ever have been designed by Providence as an evil to mankind. (Swift)

It is as natural for man to die, as to be born; and to the little infant, perhaps the one is as painful as the other. (Bacon)

Death is the golden key that opens the palace of eternity. (Milton)

It is not death, it is dying that alarms me. (Montaigne)

Ah! what a sign it is of evil life, when death's approach is seen so terrible. (Shakespeare)

Be of good cheer about death, and know this of a truth, that no evil can happen to a good man, either in life or after death. (Socrates)

Such thoughts of beauty and sentiment, belief, fear, reproach and hope belong to Man's greatest literary imaginations; and yet, when the time of death approaches, people usually prefer old age to death. Simone de Beauvoir (1977) wrote, 'We must stop cheating: the whole meaning of our life is in question in the future that is waiting for us'. Paul Tillich (1969) claimed that, 'Since every day a little of our life is taken from us — since we are dying every day — the final hour when we cease to exist does not of itself bring death; it merely completes the death process. The horrors connected with it are a matter of imagination'.

For our purposes, it is intended to view dying as a terminal phase of life resulting from any killing disease, including injury, and to present an overview, based on social science studies, of the feelings of ordinary people suffering their dying.

Castles and Murray (1979) described two general concepts that can be identified in studies concerned with dying. First, a concept that presents the institution as being of primary importance, with dying behaviour based on the quality of the patient's interactions with environmental factors and care givers. The second concept suggests that the style of dying is inherent in the style of living, and attitudes toward death are based on whatever systems of belief and emotional strengths are brought to the task of dying. They claim that, 'These concepts are not mutually exclusive, and may be considered as dominant factors rather than sole conceptual frameworks'.

Many authors suggest that the main concern of the sufferer is not with death, but with loss of control, and helplessness, uncertainty, separation and loneliness. In *The Dying Patient* (Twycross 1975), the following poem written by a terminally ill patient illustrates these fears:

I huddle warm inside my corner bed,
Watching the other patients sipping tea.
I wonder why I'm so long getting well,
And why it is no one will talk to me.

The nurses are so kind. They brush my hair
On days I feel too ill to read or sew.
I smile and chat, try not to show my fear,
They cannot tell me what I want to know.

The visitors come in. I see their eyes
Become embarrassed as they pass my bed.
'What lovely flowers', they say, then hurry on
In case their faces show what can't be said.

The chaplain passes on his weekly round
With friendly smile and calm, untroubled brow.
He speaks with sincerity of Life,
I'd like to speak of Death, but don't know how.

The surgeon comes in, with student retinue,
Mutters to Sister, deaf to my silent plea.
I want to tell this dread I feel inside,
But they are all too kind to talk to me.

Sobel (1974) suggested that the early need to control the events which cause these kinds of feelings gives way to a realization that such control is out of reach. As this becomes clear the sick person suffers grief, fear and despair, as it becomes necessary to accept the reality of impending death. Studies reveal that people who had known the truth about their dying for 6 months or more suffered less emotionally than those who had just learned about their state of dying.

Sobel's description belongs to the experience of the person who awaits death through a lingering suffering. Simone de Beavoir (1977), reminds us that, '…at every period of our life its threat is there: there are times when we come very close to it and often enough it terrifies us'. Yet, according to Choron (1979):

> Those who face imminent death in a natural catastrophe or accident may experience death differently than those who linger in pain. Thoughts and feelings of beauty, sentiment, review of past life, may be experienced in rapid sequence; pleasant illusions may crowd out the horror of the reality until unconsciousness occurs. If the person is in considerable pain, he apparently does not experience fear and dies willingly.

When a person dies his family and friends suffer a loss, roughly in proportion to the quantity and quality of their relationship with him. The dying person, however, is losing relatives, friends and all significant others. Studies reveal that younger people, and parents who have young children, are more angry about and rejecting of death than older patients; because they felt they had more to lose. The greater the number of significant others, and the closer the sufferer's relationships with them, the greater the feelings of loss and grief he must suffer. However, as the dying person's condition continues he becomes more concerned with himself, and less interested in others. With the significance of others to him being gradually reduced, the anticipated loss of them is gradually reduced. Castles and Murray (1979) claimed that, 'The retraction of ego boundaries may continue to the point at which the patient no longer needs to deny or be depressed; he can then become more accepting of death'.

Having, until now, attempted to confine this chapter to research findings, I cannot resist closing this section with something that is likely to escape the scrutiny of research as we know it.

We sometimes congratulate ourselves at the moment of waking from a troubled dream; it may be so the moment after death . (Hawthorne)

Suffering and the family

So far the discussion has been concerned primarily with the patient himself, but important features of his suffering — such as helplessness, emotional and social adjustments — are somewhat similar for his family. The sufferer is helped by family and friends but laymen, well or sick, are no more medicaly competent in one case than the other. So when important illness occurs, family members suffer very difficult problems of adjustment.

Talcott Parsons (1951) claimed that '...the solidarity of the family imposes a very strong pressure on the healthy members to see that the sick one gets the best possible care. It is, indeed, very common, if not usual, for the pressure of family members to tip the balance in the admission of being sick enough to go to bed, or call a doctor, when the patient himself would tend to stand out longer'. The patient and his family may know only that he has a troublesome cough, has been losing weight, and is easily fatigued. They expect to learn about the condition, perhaps to receive advice about smoking or some type of medication, only to be told that investigations are necessary; and later, that the problem is carcinoma of the bronchus. More is known than before, but the news is devastating and hope is already destroyed. Parsons (1951) explained that the initial effect of this kind of situation is to demonstrate the impossibility of controlling things which were thought to be readily controllable: 'To expose unfavourable factors in the situation which were not previously appreciated and to show the fruitlessness of control measures in which people had previously had faith'.

Suffering for the family begins with the news of the incurability of the close relative. For a time they may hope that the diagnosis is wrong; indeed, they may reject the prognosis and deny its impact. However, as the illness continues, its effect becomes intensely felt as family members attempt to begin to share the feelings of their sick one. Such feelings will vary according to the depth of relationship between the dying person and his family; as well as the duration of the illness and the behaviour of the dying person.

The emotional problems of the family can be so severe as to make more difficulty for the health care team than the suffering of the patient. Twycross (1975) claimed that, 'Reactions vary and are hard to predict; the small, physically frail woman may be a tower of strength, while the tough "he-man" finds himself unable to cope'. Feelings of helplessness, grief, pretence and often guilt can be intense as the family relates to and tries to care for the dying member. Twycross claims that some family members are so repelled by the thought of death that they cannot face the one who is dying, and retreat into a world of their own. Others try to pressurize the family doctor into transferring the patient to hospital. Emotional problems between family members can become very difficult to cope with. For example, a young, healthy father suffering his children's reactions to the approaching death of their mother.

Family suffering can be eased by the dying behaviour of their sick member, especially through his composure and dignity. Attitudes among the family towards death will belong to whatever systems of belief and emotional strengths that are brought to the situation. However, support from the chaplain and health-care givers is usually welcome.

In social problems, when support of one member ceases to exist because of suffering other members must assume new roles and perhaps carry new responsibilities. These kinds of adjustments, often premature, can be difficult to achieve; sometimes at the expense of the dying member. Other social problems may cause the family to distance themselves from the dying relative. Castles and Murray (1979) claimed that several conditions, or social problems, may cause a premature farewell between patient and family. They cite the following conditions which may bring about such a 'social death':

1 Distress in the family, caused by seeing the suffering of the dying member, because the family prefer to remember the dying person as he was in health.
2 Realization by the patient that the family is distressed so that he withdraws to spare them suffering.
3 Rejection by the family, because the patient's overt behaviour or slowly approaching death makes them uncomfortable.

Twycross (1975) claimed that, 'Like the patient, the immediate family members need to work through denial, anger, bargaining, and depression, if they are to achieve a positive acceptance of the inevitable'.

Suffering and the care givers

The culture of care giving is the customary and traditional way of thinking and doing things which can be shared to a greater or lesser extent by all its members. It operates under special conditions within cultural and social systems and is characterized by a distinctive set of meanings, shared by groups and subgroups of people, whose forms of behaviour differ to some extent from those of wider society. Such people, the care givers, who are drawn from different health care professions, are brought together to meet the needs of sick people. Their primary function centres around a responsibility to do everything possible to ensure the complete, early and painless recovery of sick people. Consequently, function is institutionalized in terms of expectancies, which are embodied in the attitudes of the care givers and their patients. In this connection, Talcott Parsons (1951) offered a useful example when he claimed that:

> ...it should be noted that the burden the physician asks his patients and their families to assume on his advice, are often very severe. They include suffering — 'you have to get worse before you can get better' — as for instance in the case of a major surgical operation. They include the risk of death, permanent or lengthy disablement, severe financial costs and various others.

The culture of care giving assumes that the patient will be willing to cooperate in the care situation. As Parsons (1951) claimed: 'In terms of common sense, it can always be said that the patient has the obvious interest in getting well and hence should be ready to accept any measures which may prove necessary. But there is always the question, implicit or explicit, "How do I know this will do any good?" '.

This last question is a particularly important point, because the attribution by the care giver, of significances to the sick person (which derive from the patient's dependent and even hopeless state), causes special mechanisms of defence to develop, especially when the care giver fails to justify the recovery expectations of the patient.

In meeting their primary function of care giving, doctors, nurses and paramedical staff are expected to acquire, and use, technical competence in their applied science. Yet factors of known impossibility and of uncertainty in the situation with which they have to cope make it difficult for practitioners to employ a rational approach to the task of securing patient recovery. The general effect of the existence of these factors is to impose an ever-present stress on the care giver, based upon an awareness of the possibility of illness developments which fall outside their control. Without any secure guarantee of success with competence, together with personal problems concerning fallibility and emotional involvement in judgement, the elements of strain in the care-giving situation can be considerable.

Concurrent with such problems goes the problem of reciprocal interactions with their patient and the patient's family. In this regard, I have only hinted at how care givers are brought into close contact with suffering, and that they are the group to whom sick people look for support, in relation to their anxieties about illness and the possibility of death — these kinds of interactions are taken as read. However, given that care givers, despite their acquired culture and discipline of training, belong to a wider society, it would be strange if they were altogether exempted from the kinds of emotional reactions of ordinary people to illness situations. It might prove useful, therefore, to take a wider view of attitudes toward suffering and death by considering how social values, carried in personal value systems, are reflected in the responsibilities assumed by society's care givers.

For the pioneers of modern nursing, in the nineteenth century, the orientation for nursing actions centred around a threefold objective: nursing for life, nursing for death, and nursing for recovery. Children were nursed that they might grow up into good and useful men and women; old people that they might die peacefully and, as far as possible, painlessly; and sick people that they might recover if at all possible (McGilloway 1981).

The common-sense view is that the death of a child, robbed of a full life, is a far greater loss than the death of an old person. The old person deserves dignity after a full and useful life. The young adult will be missed because of his potential contribution to his society which goes unrealized. Other characteristics of social value include beauty, talent, achievement, social class and personality traits, and it can be argued that the total amount of such characteristics lost, with the death of any person, will indicate the amount of loss to society. One cannot imagine an uncomplicated view by society, including care givers, where social and personal values do not impinge in terms of hierarchies of social worth. While the primary function of care giving protects the recovery interests of all sick people, some people, when assuming patient status, are more popular than others and some deaths can undoubtedly be rationalized more easily than others.

If all these factors, which include strong pressures to involve the care giver in a personal way, are taken together, it becomes evident that the situation of care giving is such as to cause serious problems of adjustment for its practitioners. Distancing devices such as the use of jargon, social language, treatment rituals, or detached attitudes are brought into play. Such defence mechanisms permit care givers to confine reciprocal interactions to a certain content field while, at the same time, offering some protection against feelings of grief for their patient's sufferings.

The redemptive status of suffering

For some people, in certain situations, suffering is made more acceptable when considered in the context of their own religious beliefs. Social studies reveal that the great majority of dying patients seek peace with their God. In Chapter 2 I attempted to describe how the teachings of most of the major religions influence ideas about death. Here, within Christian teaching, I will stay with the general notion of suffering through illness, to consider how devout people use their illness in a redemptive way by offering their suffering bodies in union with Christ's suffering on the cross. Dalrymple (1983) explained that some writers take issue with a broadening of the idea of redemptive suffering to include not only suffering undergone in the Christian cause, but any suffering whatsoever. Myco (1983) does not accept that all suffering can be claimed to be redemptive, rather she describes levels or strata of redemption. McNutt (1977) attempted to qualify the redemptive status of sickness, when he claimed that, 'We have no record of Christ being sick. Nor do most Christians seem to feel that sickness would be appropriate to his character and mission'.

It might be helpful, in the first instance, to attempt a brief account of the tradition of redemptive suffering, to provide the relevant setting in which these viewpoints might be interpreted. It might also help us to gain insight into how suffering can, paradoxically, make the sufferer 'strong'.

The Christian religion centres around the suffering and death of Jesus of Nazareth, who is called Christ, and hence the name Christians. All Christians down through the centuries, whatever their denomination, have been united in thinking that the death of Christ was the most important single event of their religion. His suffering, and death on the cross, stand at the centre of Christian devotion, and the Cross became the symbol of Christianity. Central to the many devotions to the suffering of Christ have been beliefs that his death was for the redemption of sin; something which is difficult to comprehend, and perhaps the reason why many have placed so much emphasis on *how* Christ suffered. Believers simply accept that Christ's death was for human sin, and concentrate on the easily comprehended bodily details of his death. Christians also believe that there is a connection between Christ's suffering on the way to death and their own personal tribulations. His cross is in some way linked to the Christian's own individual 'cross'.

Present-day sufferers must link themselves with the suffering of Christ through their imagination. Early Christians did not have this problem in that their sufferings, including persecution and death, were more directly linked with the death of Christ. They knew that by becoming Christians they would be persecuted, but they rejoiced in believing that they were proving themselves worthy of following Christ's example.

The willingness of the disciples of Christ to accept persecution and torture led to the tradition of accepting suffering as a special way of being united with Christ. Many individuals across the centuries, reflecting on the words of St Paul — 'I have been crucified with Christ' — were given the strength and hope to endure great privation. The Roman Catholic church has taken and developed the idea of suffering in union with Christ a step further, by teaching that such a union is not only redemptive for the individual but for the whole, including non-Christian, world. It is believed that since Christ died to redeem the world, suffering in union with Christ can be offered up for the same purpose; for special intention within the general intention of Christ's objective of redemption for mankind.

I mentioned earlier that some authors take issue with a broadening of the idea of redemptive suffering to include any suffering whatsoever. Myco (1983) claimed that, 'When I sit in the dentist's chair, I feel I am suffering, but I could not claim that my suffering has any redemptive status. If I complain to my friends, they would dismiss my moaning with comments such as, "Your teeth are old!", or "You should look after your teeth!"'. McNutt (1977) agreed with this concept when he explained that, 'Like most things in life, pain can be helpful or harmful; its purpose is to call our attention to the afflicted part so we can remove what is hurting us. A headache in itself is not naturally helpful; it is helpful in that it indicates to me that I am harming myself in some way (like worrying too much), and that I should change my lifestyle'. Myco (1983) claimed that there are different levels or strata of redemption in suffering. She pointed out that suffering can be caused by neglect, and in some cases it can be self-inflicted, giving rise to a difference between the avoidable and unavoidable. She claimed that: 'If a 16-year-old motor cyclist becomes permanently paralyzed in an accident, the neighbours of the family might be heard to say, "How awful, but wasn't he always a bit of a tearaway?". But, when...a

young woman lies bedridden with rheumatoid arthritis, what do we say?'.
The answer might lie with McNutt (1977), who claimed that, 'Then we
have to go to another level, where we might be taught endurance or be
freed from over-reliance on the lower elements of life — to turn to God
alone.... The level of dealing with it may well help me as a person to
grow'. He goes on to explain that, 'This is God bringing higher good out of
what is evil'.

Many lay Christians, and most clergy, find difficulty viewing illness
itself as redemptive suffering; for some illness is redemptive, but not on its
own level. It is evil on the level of body experience. McNutt (1977) wrote
that '...suffering is offered to us as a concomitant to Christian vocation,
but sickness — a particular kind of suffering caused by the interior
breakdown of a human being — is not only promised, but quite the
reverse, its healing is promised'. None the less, there is always the illness
that has not been healed, and which, somehow, the patient must learn to
deal with and accept. His illness becomes redemptive when the illness
experience is raised to the 'level of the cross'. McNutt accepts that some
people will not be healed, because it is not God's will for this to happen,
and offers an explanation by claiming that, 'The tradition of saints being
called to this kind of redemptive suffering supports the fact that God does
call some people in a special way'.

The redemptive status of any illness experience, even above the level of
body experience, is challenged by those who conclude that the only
suffering a Christian can legitimately call redemptive is the suffering
which he brings upon himself by his Christian stance in public and,
perhaps, in private. Yoder, in Dalrymple (1983), offers the following:

> The cross of Christ was not an inexplicable or chance event, which happened
> to strike him, like illness or accident. To accept the cross as his destiny, to
> move towards it and even to provoke it, when he could well have done
> otherwise, was Jesus's constantly reiterated free choice; and he warns his
> disciples lest their embarking on the same path be less conscious of its costs.
> The cross of Calvary was not a difficult family situation, not a frustration of
> visions of personal fulfilment, a crushing debt, or a nagging in-law; it was the
> political, legally to be expected result of a clash with the powers ruling his
> society'.

This confines the idea of the cross to the particular and denies all sufferers
the opportunity to cope with personal hardships, like illness or disappointment, by offering them up. Dalrymple (1983) can see this point of view,

but is reluctant not to extend the idea of redemptive suffering beyond the particular to the general. He wrote:

> What makes suffering Christian, and redemptive, is not only its content (suffering in the cause of Christ), but also its agent (Christ joined to us). From the point of view of its content, perhaps only sufferings in the direct cause of the Kingdom qualify as crosses. From the point of view of who suffers, however, all hardship *can be made* Christian, and therefore redemptive, by an act of intention of joining ourselves, branch to vine, to the redeeming Christ. In that way, we can convert, if we try, all hardships which come our way into the redemptive cross of Christ, by an act of prayerful offering. To do that is to unite our sufferings with Christ at the primary level of his obedience to the Father. That was the level, after all, at which he redeemed mankind'.

Such concepts of Christian theology can be transferred into a few words from a Christian patient, who was suffering from a metastasizing cancer of the breast. Her words (in Burkitt 1976) seem a relevant way to close this chapter:

> All this suffering I share with thousands upon thousands of other people. What I should love to do is to share too something of the joy which contains it, and the great depths of peace which lie under it, like the life-giving waters that lie under the fields and woods. I am proving the truth of what Christ said to his followers, 'My own peace I give You'. This is because God in Christ has revealed Himself to me in a new way and His presence has become increasingly real to me in this suffering. Although I have for many years known something of what it means to offer my life to Christ and practise the realization of His presence, I have recently, in a new way been able to see His glory everywhere, to know Him better and to be more ready to accept His will. I know that when He said 'Happy are those who mourn, God will comfort them', He meant exactly that. And the word translated as 'comfort' does not mean make comfortable, but make strong'. What makes us strong is His presence, a presence which is here with us now, and also waiting for us on the other side of death'.

References

Burkitt, D P (1976) Our Priorities, C.M.F. publications

Burrell, Z L and Burrell, L O (1977) Critical Care, C V Mosby

Castles, M R and Murray, R B (1979) Dying in an Institution: Nurse/Patient Perspectives, Appleton-Century-Crofts

Chroron, J, in Castles, M R and Murray, R B (1979) Dying in an Institution: Nurse/Patient Perspectives, Appleton-Century-Crofts

Dalrymple, J (1983) The Cross a Pasture, Darton, Longman and Todd

de Beauvoir, S (1977) Old Age, Penguin Books

Gabriel, R (1981) Renal Medicine, Balliere Tindall

McGilloway, F A (1976) Dependency and vulnerability in the nurse/patient situation, Journal of Advanced Nursing, 1: 229–236

McGilloway, F A (1979) One aspect of the social/psychological element of the illness state, International Journal of Nursing Studies, 16: 267–273

McGilloway, F A (1981) Nursing science: an unfolding in sequence, in J P Smith (Editor) Nursing Science in Nursing Practice, Butterworths

McGilloway, F A and Donnelly, L (1977) Religion and patient care: the functionalist approach, Journal of Advanced Nursing, 2: 3-13

McNutt, F (1977) The Power to Heal, Ave Maria Press, Notre Dame

Myco, F (1983) Nursing Care of the Hemiplegic Stroke Patient, Harper and Row

Parsons, T (1951) The Social System, The Free Press

Schutz, A (1971) The stranger: an essay in social psychology, in School and Society, Open University Press

Sobel, D (1974) Dying and death, American Journal of Nursing, 74: 98

Tillich, P (1969) The Courage to Be, Collins

Twycross, R G (1975) The Dying Patient, C.M.F. Publications

Further reading

Catrevas, C N and Edwards, J (1936) The New Dictionary of Thoughts, Waverley Book Co.

Evely, L (1974) Suffering, Image Books

Linn, M J Linn, M and Linn, D (1979) Healing the Dying, Paulist Press

McNutt, F (1974) Healing, Ave Maria Press, Notre Dame

CHAPTER 5

SPIRITUAL CARE: THE POTENTIAL FOR HEALING

Introduction

> God is within us and His love is within us. As a result when we ask God to heal — and sometimes even when we don't ask, when His very presence is in itself enough to heal — He will manifest His healing power *with* and *in* and *through* us.

Written by Father Francis McNutt, the author of *Healing* (1974), a 'best seller' on the healing ministry, these words will interest any nurse concerned with the spiritual care of her patients. And in *The Power to Heal* (1977) McNutt describes how studies in the New York University School of Nursing on the effects of nurses 'laying hands' on patients, with the intention of healing, provides evidence to show that 'simply in the natural order' the patient's power of recovery improves. Yet these findings will not surprise any nurse familiar with the writings of Nightingale (1859); the sentiments of O'Neill and Barnett (1888); the very first piece of nursing research, by Peplau (1952); the work of Harmer and Henderson (1955), Orlando (1961) and Henderson (1966), or other contemporary nurse theorists. Many health care professionals accept the importance of the nurse–patient relationship as a significant therapeutic process in a psychosocial sense, but to recognize a spiritual presence in such a relationship is a matter which is open to some scepticism.

Therefore, before following this line of thought, and bearing in mind the fact that many professionals feel uncomfortable about the notion of healing through touch and prayer, it might be worth while to look at the kinds of emphases, as we understand them, within the field of health care.

Body, mind and spirit

Looking across the field of health care, there can be no doubt that the major emphasis is being placed on looking after the purely physical nature of man. Alongside this, there is a good deal of work concerning preventive care, and noteworthy advances have taken place in this sphere. But preventive care is relatively insignificant when contrasted with the development of life-support systems, the range of modern therapies and other innovations in the curative sphere. Across the field of health, we find care of the diseases of the mind doing its best to keep up with care of the diseases of the body; but progress is slow and laboured. Care of the mind takes a poor second place to providing for the body. Why mental illness, the most abstract and challenging issue in the field of health care, should hold such a position is not clear, but it does not receive appropriate attention in the order of priorities in most societies. In this connection, physician Webb-Peploe (1975) believed that glamour and excitement, and what he terms 'the lure of the spectacular', could explain the lack of attention paid to mental health. He argued that we succumb to the temptation to do something spectacular if we allow what appear to be the more mundane aspects of health care to be squeezed out by the excitement of technology. Webb-Peploe claimed that, 'This can occur on a national level — too much money to the glamourous institutions, too little to the mental hospitals and the institutions for the subnormal'.

While psychiatric care is relegated to some sort of second place, in the order of priorities, spiritual care is difficult to find. Indeed, it is viewed as something for the attention of chaplains and 'people like that' (according to a recent survey of 33 medical wards by McGilloway 1979) but not for busy doctors and nurses who do their best to keep sick people alive. In this regard, it would be wrong to criticize or attempt to disparage any genuine efforts to meet the physical needs of ailing people, if this is the extent of the individual professional's perspective; but it is difficult to be impressed by those who claim to know better, yet claim that they have too much to do to concern themselves with the spiritual care of their patients.

The term 'profession' owes its name to the vow, or profession, that a person used to make on entering a serving community. In the Western world such communities were usually Christian in origin and ethics. Originally, the nursing profession belonged to the religious orders. Concerning the present situation, Jackson (1975) has this to offer: 'Our grandfathers held to both Christian doctrine and its ethics; our fathers abandoned the doctrine, but tried to keep the ethics; as a result, we, their children, now find it hard to possess either'. Surgeon Denis Burkitt (1976) claimed that, 'So far has scientific achievement progressively taken the place of God in the Western world that man's spiritual nature has been relegated to a position of such trivial insignificance that in many circles its very existence is questioned'. If this is the prevailing perspective, it is not surprising that surgeon Douglas Jackson (1975) argued that, 'what we need as a profession today is a continuing steady feed-in of young men and women whose lives are dominated by their commitment to God'. It can be claimed that the nursing profession has profited beyond measure from its religious background; and that to fail to respond to the spirit of this heritage is to admit to a lack of insight and to serious shortcomings in our professionalism.

Having stated this, it would be wrong to view hard work and endeavour in any negative way; for example, the struggles of research to overcome cancer. Also, it would be shortsighted not to welcome advances in genetics, immunology, and neurology, to mention a few, but it is necessary to question the popular notion that health care achievement, through science and technology, is the only reliable source to which we can turn in order to solve our problems. Far too many problems associated with health care fall outside the scope of science and technology. Burkitt (1976) put forward the following argument:

> ... we are inwardly aware that many problems ... overshadowing our hospitals and troubling our homes are seldom related to academic inadequacy. They are outside the realm that is amenable to scientific exploration or even financial rescue. The basic problems are seldom deficiences in ability and resources but relate to deeper problems of attitudes and relationships. Few problems arise with regard to techniques for procuring abortion or the mechanics of initiating or terminating resuscitation. Reducing alcoholism or drug addiction involves moral, and spiritual, rather than scientific resources. Science cannot judicate in such matters; it has nothing to say on the true nature of man, the sanctity of life or moral standards... .

None the less, our undisputed pattern of emphasis is body, then mind, and, finally, spirit. These are the three dimensions which St Paul referred to, but in a different order, 'May God ... keep you sound in spirit, soul (mind), and body'. (1 Thessalonians 5:23).

The nature of man

The concepts of uncertainty or contingency, powerlessness and scarcity, belong to us all (O'Dea 1966). We live in conditions of uncertainty with all human ventures, no matter how carefully planned or expertly executed, liable to disappointment. Powerlessness is another basic feature of the human situation and refers to the fact that not everything we desire can be attained. The range of possible complexities in this connection is very great and includes suffering, risk of death, or lengthy or permanent disability (McGilloway and Donnelly 1977). To the characteristics of uncertainty and powerlessness must be added scarcity, that is the frustrations and deprivations inherent in any human existence. Life, as we understand it, exists amid conditions of scarcity, and the problem of meaning arises as to the reasoning behind this unhappy arrangement. Many health care professionals have experienced the sense of uselessness in the presence of the patient, or relative, who could not understand why 'this was happening' to them or their loved one. Pressing questions are put to nurses and doctors concerning the frustration of expectancies of things such as recovery of a normal lifestyle, or possibility of death.

Uncertainty, powerlessness and scarcity — as inherent characteristics of human nature — bring people face to face with situations in which medical science and technology fail. This is, therefore, a time when a deep understanding of man's nature, as a larger total reality becomes necessary. In the context of this larger reality the problems of sick people, and the value of spiritual care, may be seen as meaningful in an ultimate sense.

Many of the problems facing health care professionals today must be influenced by our view of the nature of man. Whether the people we care for 'are viewed as merely, or considerably more than, the most advanced form of biological existence, will inevitably affect our decisions, for example, on the justification or otherwise of a liberal abortion policy or the introduction of euthanasia'. (Burkitt 1976).

But what is man? Maconachie (1981) reflected that, 'Man, says the scientist, is a compound of organic matter and various gases. Man, says the philosopher, is a strange phenomenon who is capable of doubting the very nature of reality. Man, says the theologian, is King of God's creation. What is man?'. Scheler (1928) observed that, 'Throughout the ages, a multiplicity of sciences have come into being, which have engaged themselves in the study of man, but have tended more to confuse ... rather than to elucidate our concept of man'. Almost 50 years later, Vernon Reynolds (1976) claimed that there is no holistic approach to man; instead there are many human sciences. He wrote: 'There is human palaeontology, human genetics, human evolution, physical anthropology, social anthropology, sociology, social psychology .... What, in such circumstances, is a holistic approach to the study of man to look like?' He turns to biology for answers, but only manages to raise more questions.

The story of the Creation, in the early chapters of the Bible, portrays man as being much more than a biological creature; that his spiritual nature makes him greater than, and apart from, other animals. Basile (1976) claimed that the greatness of man is declared from the first page in the Bible, when God is held to say, 'Let us make man in our image', and this is man being bound to infinity. He further claimed that:

> If one observes the branches of the evolutionary tree, one sees all the branches spread out, bow and fall successively, while the central shoot continues growing vertically; man is the only species at present which has really progressed; all the animal species have finally stopped in a cul-de-sac. Have we arrived at a new joint in the vertical shoot where the branch — human this time — is going to lose itself God knows where?

The Catholic Nurses' Guild, Nurses' Christian Fellowship and similar associations believe that man has a spiritual dimension which provides the potential for a Godward awareness and relationship, and the message throughout the Bible is that this potential can be realized. The Reverend Douglas Pett (1973) wrote that, 'People are found naturally looking in this direction to find some sense in their suffering; to be assured of some enduring value in themselves ... and above all to discover some meaning in their existence'. Finally, one is reminded of St Paul's assertion that 'though the outward man perish, the inward man is renewed day by day', (2 Corinthians 4:16). Yet, in present-day health care, while the outward man is nurtured the inward man is largely ignored. The spiritual aspects of the sick person can only be neglected at the risk of some damage to his total integrity.

The tradition of nursing

Throughout history, from Fabiola to Madame le Gras, caring for the sick and helping the widowed, aged, orphaned and lonely were regarded as nursing duties and works of mercy. For some — for example the Sisters of Charity, founded in 1633 by St Vincent de Paul — nursing provided the means of expressing the true love of God and the true spirit of the Gospel. Two famous Irish Sisterhoods, namely the Irish Sisters of Charity and the Sisters of Mercy, along with Pastor Fleidners' Deaconesses and Elizabeth

Fry's Protestant nursing sisters, are other examples of women who achieved a high degree of sanctity through nursing. Florence Nightingale, in the second half of the nineteenth century, helped to open nursing as a career for lay women; and her own vocation enabled her to see the modern nurse as someone motivated by spiritual ideals, but whose skills belonged to sound training and science (McGilloway 1981). The writings of Nightingale mark the beginning of theoretical models in nursing, and nursing emerging as a formalized range of activities. However, Nightingale's (1859) claim that the goal of nursing is 'to put the patient in the best condition for nature to act upon him' is far from being realized; bearing in mind his total spiritual, physical and psychosocial needs. Many might argue that Nightingale could not have imagined the range of activities concerning nurses and nursing in the second half of the twentieth century, with its computers and machines, concepts and processes. However, with such age-old problems as uncertainty, powerlessness and other spiritual issues still bothering patients today we cannot begin to claim that we offer total patient care if such fundamental things are overlooked. Nurses cannot afford to deny that such problems exist, especially when they clearly fall within the scope of opportunity available to any nurse. In this connection, Pole (1964) claimed that:

> Working among the sick who are particularly impressionable, and among their relatives, who are anxious to pin their hopes on her, the nurse has a unique advantage and a unique responsibility akin to that of the doctor, but in a way more evident; her contact with the individual patient is more prolonged … and, therefore, her actions are even more open to scrutiny and question.

The special identity in nursing is the opportunity it affords to discover the less obvious needs of a sick person because, alongside what might be called a straightforward technical task, the nurse deals with people in situations which involve intimacies. She is permitted to touch the body of another, a privilege in most societies, and has access to personal information which normally might only be disclosed to a friend or close relative (McGilloway 1976). In any nurse–patient relationship, the touch of the nurse and the words which she offers to the patient can have a powerful, comforting and reassuring effect. Some authorities go so far as to claim that her touch and prayers can actually heal. Considerations, therefore, should include any special therapeutic value which might be attributed to any nurse through her touch and words.

Healing through touch and prayer

While many health care professionals feel uncomfortable about the notion of healing through touch and prayer, there are so many sincere and intelligent doctors, nurses, teachers and clergymen who do believe in these media for healing that it seems necessary to keep an open mind on the subject. One of the most famous advocates for healing through touch and prayer is Father Francis McNutt who, in his book *The Power to Heal* (1977), describes what he calls spiritual, emotional and physical healings. He claimed that:

> Many of the things I have seen are so wonderful as to sound incredible to those who have not themselves experienced them. These saving actions of God include spiritual healings (such as being freed instantly from longstanding alcoholism), emotional healings (such as release from schizophrenia and deep mental depression) and physical healing (such as growths disappearing in a matter of minutes). For some these healings are immediate; for some they are gradual and take months, and for still others nothing at all seems to happen.

McNutt claims that about 75% of the people cared for through touch and prayer, whether for physical or emotional ailments, are either healed completely or experience a noticeable improvement. The forces which bring about such healing are claimed as being manifold, but can be grouped under the following headings.

Prenatural forces

Many communities believe that evil spirits exist, and cause illness, yet also heal by removing the illness they cause. In many cultures there are witches who claim to curse and also to cure, and many ordinary people seek such traditional help. It is held to be important, therefore, to acknowledge the existence of these forces rather than to deny them. And to offer the power of God as a replacement in healing, so that sick people will not feel it necessary to seek help from their '*curandero*' whose powers could be ultimately destructive.

Purely natural forces

These are claimed to operate through several media, the most common of

which are:
1 The power of suggestion, especially when there is a strong desire for healing on the part of the sick person, coupled with a positive suggestion.
2 Christian love, which is said to have a considerable curative power of its own.
3 The laying on of hands. Turner (1978) claimed that God takes a hand wherever He can find it; for example, the hand of a mother may be used to guide her child, or the hand of a doctor may relieve pain; 'They are all hands touched by His spirit, and His spirit is everywhere looking for hands to use'.

Natural forces, but in an extraordinary manner

Sometimes an ailment, for example a tumour, will be said to have disappeared during prayer. The disappearance of the ailment can be brought about by medical means, but it has been claimed that an inoperable growth can disappear during or after prayer; sometimes in a matter of minutes.

Speeding up the natural recuperative forces of the body

This seems to be the most common type of healing by touch and prayer. McNutt (1977) wrote: Of its very nature it cannot be proven, because the cure is accomplished through the natural recuperative forces of the body. Yet, healing might not have taken place at all or might not have happened so fast, if the prayer had not somehow stimulated and quickened the sick person's body'. Regarding psychosomatic influences, because of the close interrelationship between our bodies and our emotional and spiritual health, some physical sicknesses clear up when the roots of anxiety or bitterness are removed through touch and prayer.

A creative act of God, or miracle

This type of healing, the rarest of all, is the most difficult to believe; but most people accept that something called a miracle can happen. Among the more extreme are the accounts of people who claim to have experienced the filling of dental cavities through prayer. Some people have interpreted, in a literal way, Psalm 81:10 which says, 'I am the Lord thy God, which brought thee out of the land of Egypt: open wide thy mouth, and I will fill it'. Strange as it may seem, Fry (1970) offers that there are ministers of religion who claim that, every year since 1960, over 1000 people believe their teeth have been filled during prayer, and over 100 received complete new teeth. McNutt (1974) related the story of such a claim by a woman who said:

> I went into our living room and prayed in the Spirit and took God at His word in Psalm 81:10. I hated not to trust, but I finally went into the bathroom to see, and sure enough, the Lord had filled two teeth. I knew that if God could create the earth with all its gold and silver, it wouldn't be too much to fill my teeth.

McNutt (1977) wrote, 'If all the above seems a little complicated, that's because it is often difficult to try to gain an intellectual understanding of the manifold ways in which God works'. He adds, 'I would encourage any of you who question all this ... to check it out for yourself. Healing is caused by far more than the power of suggestion or even what can be achieved through the love of a compassionate person'.

New insights into nursing practice

Maconachie (1981) claimed that, of all health professionals, nurses have the best chance to find out what help the patient wants, and that many nurses have already recognized the spiritual needs of people and the value of touch and prayer. She offers examples of seven people: patients suffering unconsciousness, renal calculi, peritonitis, otitis media, depression, grit in the eye, and cancer, who recovered through touch and prayer. Edwards (1975) claimed that many nurses and doctors possess the healing potential, even though they may not be aware of it. He explains that, 'There is a reason why patients seem to get better more easily under one nurse than another. Some patients gather strength more quickly ... when there is an affinity between the patient and a particular nurse'. Henderson (1977) wrote, '... and the more highly developed she (the nurse) is spiritually, and the broader her tolerance of all types of faith, the greater will be her service to patients'. Henderson would like the nurse to widen her knowledge of religions so that she can increase her faith and her healing power.

Kreiger (1981) described her experiments teaching nurses to lay hands on their patients with the intention of healing. Her studies indicate a possible natural power in the 'laying on of hands'; provided that the nurse has an intent to heal another, and is physically healthy herself. Kreiger believes that 'the practice of therapeutic touch is a natural potential in physically healthy persons who are strongly motivated to help ill people and that this potential can be actualized. It is argued that caring people have a natural power of life, of energy which is communicated through the power of touch, and that the body of the sick person can build up its own life forces by absorbing this energy.

Boguslawski (1979) described the study and use of touch as an empathic concern. She claimed that man has four major levels directly related to health, namely, physical, etheric (half to two inches below the physical level), emotional and mental, and that sickness is the result of disharmony of these levels with a loss of energy. Through touch the lost energy can be replaced. 'In using therapeutic touch, the nurse helps another by enhancing the innate tendency for wellness within that individual through transduction and transmission of universal, orderly healing energies' (Boguslawski 1979).

For many, this line of argument might seem a bit fanciful, while others may consider it unnecessary to have to employ jargon to attempt to explain a natural phenomenon. Edwards (1975) seems content to believe that it is the feeling of inner compassion and sympathy of the sick, a deep inner yearning to take away pain, suffering and sickness, that are the qualities required for possession of the healing gift. For me, the important issue in all of this belongs to the fact that many nurses, and doctors, can view caring as something more than treating a pathology or managing a psychosocial dilemma. And, if dedicated nurses, doctors and other carers are able to heal the sick through touch and words, or prayer, they are privileged people.

My concluding comment rests with the College of Physicians in Paris, who have printed above their portals, 'We dressed his wounds, but God healed them'.

References

Basile, J (1976) The Sacred Rights of Life, in The Service of Life, Faith, and Profession, Sixth European Regional Congress of Catholic Nurses, Dublin

Boguslawski, M (1979) The use of therapeutic touch in nursing, Continuing Education Nursing, 10: 9–15

Burkitt, D P (1976) Our Priorities, C.M.F. Publications

Edwards, H (1975) The science of spiritual healing, Nursing Times, 71: 2008–2010

Fry, D W (1970) Can God Fill Teeth? C.S.A. Press

Harmer, B and Henderson, V (1955) Textbook of the Principles and Practice of Nursing, Macmillan

Henderson, V (1966) The Nature of Nursing, Macmillan

Henderson, V (1977) Basic Principles of Nursing Care, International Council of Nurses

Jackson, D (1975) Is the Profession Losing its Soul? Some Disturbing Trends, C.M.F. Publications

Kreiger, D (1981) Foundations for Holistic Health Nursing Practice, J B Lippincott

McNutt, F (1974) Healing, Ave Maria Press, Notre Dame

McNutt, F (1977) The Power to Heal, Ave Maria Press, Notre Dame

Maconachie, C L (1981) Spiritual Healing, Unpublished dissertation, Department of Nursing, New University of Ulster

McGilloway, F A (1976) Dependency and vulnerability in the nurse–patient situation, Journal of Advanced Nursing, 1: 229–236

McGilloway, F A (1979) Care of the Elderly — a national and international issue, Journal of Advanced Nursing, 4: 545–55

McGilloway, F A (1981) Nursing Science: An Unfolding in Sequence, in J P Smith (Editor) Nursing Science in Nursing Practice, Butterworths

McGilloway, F A and Donnelly, L (1977) Religion and patient care: the functionalist approach, Journal of Advanced Nursing, 2: 3–13

Nightingale, F (1859) Notes on Nursing: What it is and What it is Not, Harrison

O'Dea, T F (1966) The Sociology of Religion, Prentice Hall

O'Neill, H C and Barnett, E A (1888) Our Nurses and the Work They Have to Do, Ward, Lock and Company

Orlando, I (1961) The Dynamic Nurse–Patient Relationship, Putnams

Peplau, H (1952) Interpersonal Relations in Nursing, Putnams

Pett, D (1973) The hospital chaplain, Nursing Times, 69: 405–406

Pole, K F M (1964) Handbook for the Catholic Nurse, Robert Hall

Reynolds, V (1976) The Biology of Human Action, W H Freeman and Co.

Scheler, M (1928) Die Stelling des Menschen in Kosmos, Interuniversity Press

Turner, J (1978) The Healing Church, Christian Journals

Webb-Peploe, M M (1975) Is the Profession Losing its Soul? Some Disturbing Trends, Chapter 1, C.M.F. Publications

PART TWO

SOME RELIGIOUS PRACTICES AND THEIR MEANING

CHAPTER 6

THE CHRISTIAN PATIENT AND THE CHAPLAIN

Introduction

Christianity has been involved with the care of the sick since its inception. One of the appeals of Jesus Christ is that he cured the sick, made the blind see, the lame walk, and brought relief to the mentally ill. One of the earliest developments of Christianity was the setting up of the diaconate, and one of their duties was to care for the sick and vulnerable. At a later date monasteries of religious men and women were established, many of which had an infirmary where the sick of the area were cared for, and this became a feature which we have come to associate in particular with the monasteries of the Middle Ages, although this religious age began much earlier.

In the present century, as well as the previous one, Christianity has demonstrated its continuing aim to care for the sick by the establishing of religious medical and nursing orders, of men and women who tend the sick, across the world. This care is offered in State hospitals as well as hospitals of the religious orders.

Fundamental questions

In the context of this chapter, emphasis is placed on the care of sick people in State hospitals, where the religious needs of the Christian patient are met by the appointment of chaplains of various denominations.

The religious needs of people are often accentuated by their stay in hospital; the patient in the bed experiences a certain amount of strain by the very fact of being ill. And he is sometimes faced with basic or fundamental questions for the first time; questions that do not have the same immediacy when he is in full health, and busying himself with everyday activities. In hospital, he may find himself wondering, 'Why am I ill?', and 'Why did this have to happen to me?', or, 'Am I going to recover?', or, 'Are they hiding something from me?'. It is questions such as these that the chaplain has to try to answer. The questions, 'Why am I ill?', and 'Why did this have to happen to me?', are philosophical and religious questions. They raise the whole problem of illness and evil. Why is there evil and suffering in this world? Why do we have to weaken and die? Why, if God is so good, did He create these kinds of things? Dealing with questions like these requires time and patience from the chaplain, who attempts to enable the sufferer to understand that we have to live in this type of world; a world that is far from being ideal. The chaplain will point out that Christ accepted the world as it is, and answered the questions of man in a particular way. Christians believe that Christ died on the cross and arose from the dead to redeem man from the penalty of sin, and through this belief, man is offered the opportunity to unite his own suffering with the death and resurrection of Christ, to make reparation for his own sins, which are believed to be the greatest of all evils.

The other questions, 'Am I going to recover?', and 'Are they hiding something from me?', are questions which the patient may find difficult to put to the clinical members of the health care team. It is my experience that the Christian patient expects a high degree of confidence from his clergyman, and will feel more at ease bringing his anxieties to the attention of the chaplain, than to anyone else. The patient may feel unsure about his troubles, and take care not to bother highly trained doctors and nurses whom he does not know very well. He may think that his feelings of anxiety may turn out to be unimportant when so much is happening all around him in the hospital ward. He may decide that the doctors and nurses are too busy to deal with something which, at the end of the day, may have no substance. Most patients view their doctors and nurses with much respect and, sadly, it is possible for clinical staff to convey to the patient the image that they will not tolerate 'foolishness'. So it is to the chaplain that the patient will often turn, with statements such as, 'I don't know what is wrong with me', or 'I cannot understand the jargon', or, 'I think I must be dying of cancer because they keep avoiding any discussion with me'.

Coping with the answers

The important thing for the chaplain is to listen to these statements of fear.

By talking to the chaplain, the patient may be getting the first opportunity to put his anxious feelings into words. By trying to explain his fears in words, the patient may see for himself that his fears are groundless, and by providing a listening ear the chaplain may have brought relief and reassurance to the patient. The chaplain too may be guilty of giving the impression that he has not time to spend half an hour listening, but the good chaplain will have the art of being a good listener.

Yet feelings of anxiety for the patient may not be lessened by finding someone who will listen. The patient may rightly suspect that something is seriously wrong, and he is finding that the answers he is getting from different quarters are very vague. Consequently, the chaplain can sometimes find himself in a difficult situation when attempting to allay anxieties; in fact he may find himself in an invidious situation. For example, he may have learned from a relative of the patient, or a junior nurse, that the patient is in fact terminally ill. The knowledge the chaplain carries about the patient may not therefore be first-hand knowledge, in that it may not come from the doctor, or the nurse in charge of the ward. If the information comes from a family member, it will often be accompanied by a frenzied plea that the patient must not be told about the seriousness of his condition. This is a very natural reaction from a close relative who has just heard shattering news, and is not yet prepared to face the kind of relationship that will arise when both of them (relative and sick person) know that death is the outcome of the illness. The chaplain is very reluctant to initiate this new relationship and, indeed, is not empowered to do so by the ethics of his creed. As a clergyman, he cannot share information gained by hearsay, he can only do so when the doctor or nurse in charge asks him to help. In my experience as a hospital chaplain, I can only call to mind one occasion when clinical staff asked me to tell a patient about the seriousness of his condition. This is, arguably, not so important, as the major function of the chaplain is to help people cope with suffering and dying, not to make known medical outcomes. On the one occasion mentioned above, I intervened at the request of a concerned Christian surgeon who thought that one of his patients did not appreciate the seriousness of his condition. The surgeon asked me to make known to the patient that his illness was incurable. I did this, and the patient was shattered. His will to live seemed to leave him, and he died within a fortnight of receiving the news. I have often wondered if the patient's death had been hastened by the news; still I wonder.

The other side of the story can seem equally brutal at times. A young man of about 20 years of age was terminally ill; and in a close community, such as we have in rural Ireland, this fact was soon common knowledge to all except the young man. He showed no signs of anxiety until some of his peer group visited him and told him, 'We heard you were dying and came to see you'. I plead that this dilemma as to whether the patient should be told be given more consideration that it seems to receive. I will put it this way; it may happen that a terminally ill patient may have a considerable material estate to dispose of, and he has not yet made a will. In this situation, the patient will usually be told so that he may put his affairs in order. It may sometimes happen that a patient without a material estate will not be told. Keeping this in mind, it may also happen that any patient may not be spiritually prepared for death. For the Christian, to be spiritually prepared for death is more important than the wealth he may leave behind him. It is important therefore that health carers be aware of these sensitivities. Manuals of medicine say that a patient who is terminally ill, and is not spiritually prepared for death, should be told about his condition, so that he may have an opportunity, which he may or may not decide to take, to prepare himself to meet the judgement of God. The same manuals say that a patient who has material property to dispose of should also be told of his imminent death. Those who are both materially and spiritually prepared, however, need not be told of their imminent death, if prudent judgement decides that such information would impose an undue burden of suffering. Perhaps an argument can be made for consultation about the matter, between the doctor, nurse in charge and chaplain, when the latter feels that he has to face a terminally ill patient who is not spiritually prepared for death. The chaplain, in justice, cannot take it upon himself to tell the patient. He is not the person who has made the diagnosis, and his information about the situation remains hearsay until confirmed by the competent authority. To pass on information to the patient before the competent authority has requested that this should be done, would, and rightly so, lay the chaplain open to the charge that he was not working in a manner suited to the overall good of the patient.

The chaplain–patient relationship

Because of the Christian patient's evaluation of the role of the chaplain, details of his private life may be revealed to the minister; details which, in turn, he may not reveal to any other member of the health care team. These are confessional secrets and are revealed to the chaplain because, in the eyes of the patient, the chaplain is the man of God especially equipped to deal with these matters. On most occasions the confidences are of a spiritual nature, and of relevance to no one except the patient and his chaplain. However, on the odd occasion, something may be revealed to the chaplain which pertains to the patient's medical condition. It may be something which the patient is unwilling to reveal to the nurse or doctor for fear of embarrassment. If this is the case, it will be the role of the chaplain to persuade the patient that his feelings of embarrassment must be weighed against the benefit to his health, if the problem were made known to those who can deal with it. The chaplain will attempt to explain to the patient that the health care team are also used to dealing with secrets in an ethical manner and that his reticence will cause no surprise or morbid curiosity. He will try to assure the patient that medical and nursing people are dealing with such sensitive information nearly every day. The reluctant patient may ask the chaplain to reveal the information for him, and only then can the chaplain do so. If all persuasion fails, the chaplain must respect, absolutely, the confidence he has received, and to reveal such information would diminish the chaplain–patient relationship.

The chaplain's work

Chaplains of different denominations may place stress on different aspects of Christianity, but all are likely to agree that people who are sick or dying should be given the opportunity to ask for the support of their chaplain in preparation for death. And that after death the person should be treated with dignity and in the ways of his faith. Some Christian religions are less ritualistic in the ministry than others; some may stress the ministry of the 'Word' while others stress the 'Sacrament'. The Roman Catholic Church does stress the Sacrament and, for example, would normally expect a priest to be called to a very ill or dying patient. The wise thing to do is to consult with the patient and his relatives regarding the chaplain of their denomination. Most patients benefit from the attendance of their chaplain.

The Sacrament, as is proposed in the Roman Catholic ritual for the care of the sick, must be administered in a meaningful and caring manner. Formerly termed the 'Last Sacrament' the Sacrament of the Sick is administered to patients who need not be dying. It gives the sufferer and his family strength and reassurance since it is not just a preparation for death, it can be administered more than once. The Sacrament of the Sick will be discussed in a later section.

Sometimes it is difficult for the chaplain to do the job he has to do, and I would like to draw attention to one example where more thought should be given to the role of the chaplain. I think here about the patient suffering cardiac arrest. The scene to which the chaplain is called is one of great activity, with five or six practitioners around the patient trying to revive him. The chaplain often has to jostle around the bed to find a space in order to administer the last rites to the patient. It is a long-standing custom in the Roman Catholic church that a prayer should be whispered in the dying person's ear at this time. However, because of all the clinical activity at the time of the cardiac arrest it may not be possible to get near the patient. If some highly competent, and successful, doctors and nurses can carry out resuscitation and yet involve the chaplain, why cannot others? Some thought should be given to the actual mechanics of allowing the chaplain access to the patient without impeding other essential services. The most important person for the Christian patient who is going to die is, after all, his chaplain.

Those patients preparing for operation should be given an opportunity to see the chaplain. If an anaesthetic is to be administered, this meeting should take place before the patient is sedated. It can be argued that no operation is a minor one as far as the patient is concerned. It is the chaplain's role to prepare the patient spiritually for the operation by prayer, word and sacrament. This will allow the patient to face the operation reasonably happy that he is prepared for death, perchance it should occur. Such preparation is important for all Christians, whether Protestant or Roman Catholic.

If a new baby is likely to die, he or she will have to be baptized. Although the chaplain should be sent for, the baby will be baptized by a nurse who pours water over the baby's head, using the child's name and saying, 'I baptize you in the Name of the Father, and of the Son, and of the Holy Spirit'.

For some denominations of the Christian faith, certain medical and operative procedures are considered to be immoral. One difficult case is the Jehovah's Witness, whose faith requires abstinence from blood. Another difficult case for the mainstream Christian is the sterilization of a woman immediately after the birth of her baby. In the final days of pregnancy, an expectant mother may be placed in a tug-of-war situation between the doctor who is strongly advising the operation for the sake of the health of the woman, and the chaplain who is strongly pointing out its immorality. The question then becomes, 'What is good medical and psychological care in this situation?'. The answer is not immediately available, especially if it results in the patient needing psychiatric care for guilt feelings after having accepted the doctor's advice.

An interesting footnote to this section on the work of the chaplain is the control that the patient himself has in his relationship with the ministry. The patient is not normally asked if he would like to see the doctor, or the physiotherapist, when this is deemed necessary. He is, however, asked if he would like to see the chaplain; for example, before an operation. On the one hand, if the answer is no, only an insensitive chaplain would intrude; but on the other, it is unthinkable that a nurse would not pass on a patient's request to see the chaplain.

The relatives of the patient

The chaplain will be involved in various ways with the relatives of patients. Sometimes his involvement will be little more than social; for example, meeting relatives at the bedside of a patient who is not seriously ill. When the patient is ill, the chaplain's role will be to reassure them that the very best is being done for their loved one. If relatives have received assurances from the doctor, or nurse, that there is a well-founded hope for full or partial recovery, it is the chaplain's job to back up these assurances, and to ask the relatives to put their trust in the hopes of experts. In the situation of the terminally ill patient, the chaplain will help the relatives, in faith, to resign themselves to this fact, and to ask them to think of the role they can play in helping the dying person to be in a fit state to face the judgement of God. If relatives can face the imminent death of their loved one, in a spirit of faith, it helps them to cope with the fact of death when it occurs. Finally, the chaplain may be involved in some grief counselling of the relatives after the occurrence of death. This will be brief, because the chaplain will only be in touch with the relatives for about an hour after the death, yet it will lay the foundations for further counselling by the relatives' own clergyman, or some other suitably qualified person.

To conclude this section, let me venture some support for nursing staff regarding restricted visiting. By restricted visiting I mean limiting the number of people round the sick bed at any one time. When I find nurses having difficulty in applying this rule, I always do my best to support them. I do so because of my experience as a patient recovering from a minor operation. On one occasion, I had 14 visitors round my bed at the same time. The sun was shining strongly through the windows of the very crowded room, and I remember that visit as one of the most uncomfortable periods I have ever endured. I remember perspiring embarrassingly as the minutes dragged by. In short, the wisdom of having only two visitors at a time, in the interest of the patient, was easily accepted by me from then onwards.

The nurse and the Sacrament of the Sick

Apart from the Sacrament of Baptism, already mentioned, the nurse will be concerned with the Sacrament of the Eucharist (Holy Communion), and with the Sacrament of the Sick. Formerly called the Last Sacraments or 'Last Rites', the Sacrament of the Sick usually comprises Confession, Holy Communion and the Anointing with Oil. Holy Communion is regularly brought to those patients who would like to receive it. However, more people than before, who receive professional nursing care, are receiving the Sacrament of the Sick and nurses are assisting priests more often. For this reason, it may be helpful to say something about the role of the nurse regarding the part she can play in all of this. But, before that, it must be realized that at times improvisation will be necessary. In an emergency, Sacraments may be administered in any place and under any circumstances. Also, different chaplains and patients will have different needs, but the following information may prove to be helpful.

A steady table at the foot of the bed or to the side, where the patient can see it, is necessary. On the table is placed a crucifix with a candle on either side. A bottle of holy water, or a bowl with holy water, is placed in one of the front corners of the table. In the other front corner is placed a glass of drinking water. There needs to be space in the middle of the table for the priest to unfold and spread the Corporal. Some nurses also place a vase of flowers on the table.

If the Anointing with Oil is to be administered, a small dish holding cotton-wool balls (preferably six) will be needed. And another dish in which to place them after use. If possible the patient is best propped up and a napkin on his chest is helpful.

If the patient wishes to confess, the nurse and relatives will be expected to leave the room or beyond hearing distance. After the Confession and Communion, the priest will then rinse the fingers in which he held the Host in the glass of water. The patient may be offered some of this water to drink after receiving Communion. The remaining water should be poured over a plant.

The Anointing with Oil can be administered separately or immediately following Communion. The preparation already described for Holy Communion is all that is required, except that the nurse will help by removing the patient's bed socks.

The chaplain will anoint the patient with holy oil. The chaplain will have brought this oil with him. First he anoints the eyelids, then the ears, the nostrils, the lips, the palms of the hands (the back of the hands in priests), and the instep of the feet.

During this, the nurse can be very helpful by positioning or supporting the patient's head, by uncovering the patient's hands and feet and covering them again, and by handing the priest the things he may need.

After the anointing, the priest will cleanse the part anointed with a piece of cotton wool. He will then replace the holy oil in its container and, probably, take the cotton wool away with him to dispose of later.

In an emergency case, when life is hurrying away, it will suffice to have only one of the senses, or the forehead, anointed.

The chaplain–nurse relationship

The chaplain will be involved in the spiritual affairs of the Christian nurse, as well as the patient. First of all, there will be the matter of arranging church services on Sundays, to suit the main body of hospital staff. Sometimes the chaplain will be approached by a nurse about the details of Church law regarding a forthcoming marriage, or a nurse may reveal at a quiet moment many of the problems of his or her personal life that affect the quality of nursing. Many young adults who are nursing dying people, perhaps for the first time, will seek spiritual guidance and support, and they may ask the chaplain important questions about suffering and death. The chaplain may occasionally meet a particularly sensitive nurse who has feelings of doubt about self-worth, because a patient in the nurse's care died suddenly or unexpectedly. It will be the chaplain's task to assuage these feelings of guilt, especially when no blame can be attached to the nurse, and to build up his or her confidence. The presence of such feelings reveal a deeply caring person. Finally, if the chaplain finds a nurse under undue pressure from fractious relatives, he will attempt to relieve this pressure by speaking on behalf of the nurse, by giving an explanation of the many tasks and responsibilities which have to be carried out, and by asking the relatives for greater understanding.

Concluding comment

The source material for this chapter has been the writer's own observations as a hospital chaplain; the Gospel of St Luke; the Acts of the Apostles; the Roman Catholic Ritual on the care of the sick, and dying, and an article in the *Journal of Advanced Nursing*, (McGilloway and Donnelly 1977). In this article it was stated, '...it is tempting to say that many of us do not yet appreciate the importance of the spiritual needs of the ordinary ill person in a hospital bed. We are certainly uninformed....' For me, the purpose of this chapter has been to attempt to continue the process of informing, started in that article.

Reference

McGilloway, F A and Donnelly, L (1977) Religion and patient care: the functionalist approach, Journal of Advanced Nursing, 2: 3–13

CHAPTER 7

THE JEWISH PERSPECTIVE

Judaism is a religion with a strong, almost overriding, life-affirming principle. The religious principle of '*pikkuach nefesh*', the saving of life, and all the treatments associated with that aim figures prominently in all Jewish literature, and in order to save life the individual may, if necessary, transgress and forego all but three of the main commandments and prohibitions of Jewish law. The three exceptions are the prohibitions on murder, incest and idolatry. With that strong theme running through religion, it is clear that Jewish patients will, in most cases, cooperate with all forms of treatment and therapy, however unpleasant.

Much help can be given to Jewish patients by those caring for them. In order to provide this help, the nursing staff need to have a basic awareness of Jewish rituals and observances, and some understanding of the life-affirming philosophy of Judaism. They need, too, to consult the patient's family, since degrees of Jewish observance vary enormously within the Jewish population of the United Kingdom, and sometimes needless offence can be given by assuming a degree of religious observance not, in fact, present in that particular family.

Times and seasons

The Jewish calendar is a lunar one, which makes it impossible to give exact dates for the festivals since they move around within a few weeks. There is an adjustment to the solar calendar (an extra month is inserted seven times in every 19 years) which stops festivals moving right round the year. As a result one can say that Jewish New Year (Rosh Hashanah) is always in September or October and Passover (Pesach) always in March or April.

The Sabbath

The Jewish sabbath runs from sundown on Friday night until sundown (the point at which there are three stars in the sky) on Saturday evening. It is celebrated in a variety of ways by Jews. Chiefly it is a day of rest (*Shabbat*), based on two concepts out of the two versions of the Ten Commandments (Exodus 20 and Deuteronomy 5). According to Exodus God rested on the seventh day and made it holy (as in the Creation story in Genesis 1–2), and hence human beings should imitate God and do the same. The second idea is more ethically based — the Israelites were slaves in Egypt, and thus know the feelings of those who have to work all the time. For that reason the Israelites were to have a day of rest, as were any non-Israelites who worked for them, and any servants, slaves and animals.

In a very characteristic manner, the rabbis who codified much of Judaism (in the Mishnah and Talmud from about AD 200–500) tried to define what this work was which should not be carried out on the Sabbath. They came up with 39 classes of forbidden work — including, for instance, sowing, planting and lighting a fire. But associated with them and derived from them are a variety of other Sabbath prohibitions which orthodox Jews observe. These include cooking, writing, driving and handling money. Most of these would apply in hospital just as much as outside. Indeed, orthodox Jews would try hard to maintain all the Sabbath laws unless any of them actually impinged on their health.

Both orthodox and progressive (I use the term progressive to include both Liberal and Reform, and to some extent the American Conservatives) Jews would want to read for themselves or even, if it is available, attend Sabbath services. Many Jews will come to hospital with a prayerbook, but if they have not brought one the visiting rabbi or lay visitor can usually arrange for one to be brought. Two ceremonies that are very important at the beginning of the Sabbath are Kiddush, the sanctification of the Sabbath which includes a blessing over wine and is followed by a blessing over bread, and the blessing of children. Both of these are hard for staff in hospitals to arrange, but if some encouragement can be given to families to gather round their sick members on Friday evening, to create something of a Sabbath atmosphere, it can be enormously helpful. Although it is customary to say the blessing over wine, if wine of any kind were considered harmful it could easily be over grape-juice. And although the bread over which the blessing is said is usually two plaited loaves covered in poppy-seed, any bread will do — and the courtesy of bringing bread for this purpose to the bedside would be enormously appreciated by Jewish patients who normally observe these rituals at home.

One other way in which the Sabbath is often observed by Jews is by some kind of studying. In orthodox circles, this would tend to apply mostly to men. In progressive circles it could be true of either sex. In any case, nursing staff should not be surprised to discover a Jewish patient, however sick, poring over a text on the Sabbath (Saturday), as well as making *Kiddush* (blessings over wine and bread) and saying prayers.

Although Sabbath laws can be broken for the preservation of life — and one of the classic examples always given is the lighting of a fire in the sickroom — many Jews will nevertheless try to observe the Sabbath in some way whilst in hospital. Many Jews of whatever persuasion might be particularly keen to have a better meal on Friday evening — the traditionally festive Sabbath meal — and be grateful if their families were encouraged to bring in some delicacy on that day.

Rosh Hashanah — New Year

The Jewish New Year begins in the autumn, in September or October. Unlike most religions, it is not a time of rejoicing, but rather the beginning of a season of meditation and penitence. The 10 days between New Year and the Day of Atonement (Yom Kippur) are called the Ten Days of Repentance, and are used by Jews to make their apologies to fellow human beings whom they have in some way wronged over the past year. New Year itself is therefore a solemn day, with certain important customs and traditions which a Jewish patient might well wish to observe.

The first is hearing the note of the *shofar*, the ram's horn. Very often a local rabbi will willingly come in with a *shofar* and blow it for the Jewish patient (and all surrounding people!) to hear. Unless the noise itself is likely to be particularly disturbing to any of the patients in the ward — and many would find it fascinating if it were explained — this can be of enormous value to the Jewish patient. This is partly an emotional benefit — for the patient will feel remembered and cherished by the Jewish community on this particular day. But it has another less easily explicable virtue, which is, as far as it can be assessed at all, something to do with the hope of survival for another whole year. In order to justify this assertion, one of the traditional beliefs associated with Rosh Hashanah needs to be explained. According to legend (and the belief is borne out in the liturgy for New Year and the Day of Atonement), God keeps a Book of Life, in which are inscribed the names of those who will live until the next New Year. The initial verdict is given on Rosh Hashanah, but it is sealed on the Day of Atonement, which means that in the Ten Days of Repentance, 'repentance, prayer and charity can avert the severity of the decree' (an extract from a medieval prayer attributed to Rabbi Amnon of Mayence, entitled *Unnetaneh Tokef*). Although few Jews in modern times, whether orthodox or progressive, would believe this in literal terms, nevertheless New Year and the Day of Atonement have become inextricably linked with the idea of a decision being taken 'on high' as to who shall live and who die. For those who are seriously ill, therefore, it is very important that some attention is paid to their needs in these 10 days, and that they are encouraged to hear the ram's horn (*shofar*) and to apologize to those whom they feel they have wronged or offended.

In many cases, the family will take over responsibility for this. But there will undoubtedly be a fair number of Jewish patients who have no family, or whose family is distant, or whose family is totally unobservant — even sometimes impatient and disapproving. These patients need all the support and kindness they can get at this time of the year. Even those who cannot rationalize it at all will often have a deep spiritual need — a need to pray, to ask for God's forgiveness and to apologize to fellow human beings. This desire, if unrecognized, can be turned to a considerable sense of despair.

One other, less important, custom for Rosh Hashanah which may be worth mentioning is the tradition of eating apple dipped in honey to symbolize a sweet new year. Once again, the very attentiveness which makes such an observance possible for a Jewish patient is enormously appreciated — and may, indeed, contribute to a sense of being accepted in a ward which is unlikely to have an enormous number of Jews in it.

The Day of Atonement — Yom Kippur

Yom Kippur follows 10 days after Rosh Hashanah. It poses almost insuperable problems in its observance in hospital, since it is a whole day of fasting (total abstinence from food, drink, washing, brushing teeth and general grooming) and praying. The principle underlying this is that of 'affliction', that one *should* suffer on this holiest of holy days, and that although the suffering should not be unbearable, it should undoubtedly hurt. In many cases, such behaviour on the part of sick patients in hospital would be, to say the least, foolish. However, the principle of *'pikkuach nefesh'*, — the 'saving of life' — as discussed earlier, applies here. For if it would be considered dangerous even to a very minimal extent for a patient to fast (and one can imagine few situations where medical opinion would advocate fasting after surgery, for instance), then the commandment of fasting is overriden by the even greater commandment to save life.

Praying all day in bed in hospital is also not that easy to achieve. Many patients who are well enough to be up and about at least part of the day might well appreciate enormously the provision of a side-ward or a small office in which they could be quiet and meditate. If there were more than one Jew in the hospital at the time, it might also be helpful for encouragement to be given to them to hold some form of service together — even if it were fairly brief and in less than suitable surroundings. For even the least observant of Jews tend to observe Yom Kippur in some way, and there can be a considerable amount of guilt expressed, or, even worse, suppressed, over this whole penitential period. Whilst most Jews would accept that it might not be in their interests, medically speaking, to fast, they might well find it extremely difficult to let Yom Kippur pass them by without paying it any attention at all.

Sukkot — Tabernacles and Simchat Torah — the Rejoicing of the Law

Exactly 2 weeks after New Year comes Tabernacles and a week after that the Rejoicing of the Law (for Progressive Jews, whilst Orthodox Jews have the Eighth Day of Solemn Assembly, followed the next day by the Rejoicing of the Law). In most ways, patients in hospital will be unable to celebrate this festival properly. Its main features consist of the building of temporary huts, partly open to the sky, filled with fruit and flowers and covered with leafy branches. This is supposedly in memory of the temporary dwellings in which the Israelites lived when journeying across the wilderness. Associated with these temporary huts (*sukkot* — the singular form is a *sukkah*) is a strong tradition of hospitality, inviting guests to share the beauty of the *sukkah* and the plenty of the harvest. In more recent times, the festival has been an occasion for the distribution of gifts of fruit and food to elderly and needy people in the area, in a similar way to many churches' harvest festivals.

The one aspect of Sukkot which could be practised in hospital if requested is the bringing in of a particular symbol, the *lulav*. This is a palm-branch, bound together with willow twigs and myrtle shoots and held with a citron (Hebrew *etrog*) in the other hand. This goes back to a biblical injunction to celebrate the festival of Sukkot with these magnificent and beautiful branches and fruit, and, though we do not know exactly how they were used in early Temple and pre-Temple worship, in modern synagogues they are waved. This can often be arranged through a local synagogue, and may be of some comfort in giving the individual the feeling that he is carrying out as many of the religious duties (*mitzvot*) incumbent on him as he can.

The Rejoicing of the Law is a joyful festival when the scroll of the Law (the *Torah*, which consists of the five books of Moses from Genesis to Deuteronomy) is completed and rolled right back and begun again. In the synagogue there are processions and scrolls are carried around. There is singing and dancing, and the children are given apples, sweets and flags. There is no means by which quite this atmosphere can be transferred to a hospital ward. Nevertheless, the children or grandchildren of the patient can be encouraged to come in to the hospital immediately after the service, whilst the excitement is still with them, and tell of all that took place.

Chanukkah — the Festival of Light

Chanukkah is really a minor festival, which has become much more emphasized in Europe because of its close proximity to Christmas. It celebrates the victory of the Maccabees over the Seleucid Greeks (as recounted in the Apocrypha) in the second century BC. But the legend that leads to the lights is that after driving the Greeks out of the Temple, the Jews found that there was no oil to keep the eternal lamp burning — just about enough for one day. So a horseman was sent to fetch more, and by a miracle the tiny supply lasted for 8 days. As a result a Chanukkah lamp (the *Chanukkah menorah* or *chanukkiyah*) is lit, one candle on the first night, two on the second, and so on for 8 days. Some patients may wish to do this in hospital, and should be encouraged to carry out the custom if they can.

Purim

In the early spring (usually March) there is a carnival-type festival called Purim, which will hardly be celebrated by Jews in hospital. It commemorates the story of the book of Esther in the Bible and involves a lot of play acting, some noisy reading and cheering, the eating of a particular sweet cake stuffed with poppy seeds called *Hamantaschen* (Haman's ears — Haman is the villain of the story), dressing up in fancy dress and so on. The only likely celebration of the festival in hospital is the bringing of *Hamantaschen* for the patient. It is one of the jolliest of the Jewish festivals, however, and if the family can be persuaded in any way to mark it specially for the patient it could be of enormous help in lifting his or her spirits.

Passover — Pesach

This is perhaps one of the best known of all the Jewish festivals, and one of those in which nursing staff can be most helpful. Passover commemorates the journey of the Israelites from slavery in Egypt to freedom in the Promised Land. It is marked in Jewish homes by a '*seder*', a special service around the table, with a festive meal and the eating of symbolic foods. Once again, even the least observant of Jews tend to observe Passover in some way, so that in hospital almost all Jews would tend to wish the seven (eight for orthodox Jews) days of Passover to be marked out in some way.

One of the key observances of Passover is not eating leavened bread (or leaven in general). This goes back to the Exodus story in which the Israelites apparently left Egypt in such a hurry that they did not have time to let their bread rise — as a result Jews are supposed to remember this by eating unleavened bread during the 7 days of Passover. This unleavened bread is called '*matzah*' and is reasonably freely available in cities in the UK. But as well as *matzah*, the observant Jew will probably eat no leaven and nothing with normal flour in it during Passover (e.g. biscuits, cake, breakfast cereals, etc.) An orthodox Jew is so careful about what he or she eats during Passover that an ordinary hospital kitchen would find it impossible to cater. In London, the Kosher Meals Service would provide food. In many provincial cities, the local Jewish communities would help, and in most cases the family would provide the necessary food.

At this point it is important to stress that the strictness of observance of the dietary laws in general and the Passover food laws in particular does vary considerably, so that it is difficult to give a firm ruling. What is always helpful is an awareness by those caring for the patient that what he or she eats is important in more than the purely nourishing sense. Food plays an important part in Judaism — whether as a symbol, such as unleavened bread, or as a celebration, such as the enormously fattening and delicious potato pancakes *(latkes)* at Chanukkah, or as a seasonal mark, such as dairy products at Shavuot (Pentecost).

The relevance of food to individual well-being is great in all cultures, but perhaps stressed more in Judaism. Although the observance of dietary laws in general does vary considerably, Orthodox Jews do not eat pork or its products. They eat the meat of animals such as cows and sheep: only those animals that chew their cud and have cleft hooves. They also eat game birds and fishes that have scales and fins; not shellfish. The beef animals have to be slaughtered in a special manner, designed to kill them quickly and, as far as possible, painlessly. The meat is freed from blood before it is eaten. Many foods forbidden to Jews come from predatory birds or animals. Also, milk and meat products are kept apart and not served at the same meal.

There is a huge fund of jokes about Jewish mothers and their constant supply of chicken soup, a better cure than any antibiotic/bandage/operation. Despite this being obvious nonsense, food is more than usually an expression of love amongst Jews — it is considered that gifts of food at life crises are of prime importance (such as cakes brought to a house of mourning) and the preparation of chicken soup for a patient in hospital would not be at all unusual.

Pentecost — Shavuot

Fifty days after Pentecost comes Shavuot. It is a harvest festival which primarily commemorates the giving of the law to Moses on Mount Sinai. Its traditions are many — the decoration of synagogues and homes (and hospital bedsides) with flowers, the eating of fruit and dairy products, particularly amongst European Jews, cheesecake, and a long study session, in some communities all night.

The attitude to death

So much for the Sabbath and festivals. Without a little awareness of their customs, it is hard to offer extra help and comfort. But there are other areas where some knowledge can be helpful. Foremost amongst these is the attitude to death. Judaism, as already stated, is an enormously life-affirming religion, and there has been considerable unwillingness on the part of families and Jewish doctors to admit to a dying person that he or she is in fact dying. That is gradually changing, just as it is amongst other religious groups, but the huge emphasis on life-saving can mean that the patient who is clearly not going to survive gets less than his or her fair share of attention, a problem whose existence is only just being realized in the Jewish community.

This is also partly due to a very different attitude to life after death and the next world from that expressed in mainstream Christianity. Orthodox Jews assert their belief in a world to come (which is ill defined) and in physical resurrection when the Messiah comes. Progressive Jews (and a lot of orthodox Jews in private discussion) are less than certain about life after death and a 'world to come', and tend to regard immortality as a condition of the spirit, or even as the memory one leaves behind with those who carry on living. This results in a general sense that what one does in this life is what really matters, that there is no special 'salvation' in the next life if it exists, and an extraordinary practicality which asserts that since it is impossible to find out what happens in the next world, and after death, one should not bother about it but concentrate hard on this life, savouring every moment of it, up until its very end. This is crucial, for it must be a good argument for the sort of pain control piloted by the hospice movement and now in more general use, which encourages pain relief on demand and the use, as near to normally as possible, of every moment of this life here on Earth.

So for Jewish patients, the use of last days on this Earth is to be treasured and enjoyed. Despite the sadness at parting from loved ones, the grieving can only form a part of the activity of the last days — patients should be encouraged to remember the happy times and to look back to the achievements, and even to carry out one or two more last tasks, where possible. (One member of my congregation wrote a fairly irate letter to the *Daily Telegraph* on the day he died, which was published, rather fittingly, on the day of his funeral.) A combination of this, and some prayers and a silent personal confession, if wished for, create a sense of readiness, even if much is left undone.

After a Jewish patient dies, it is usual in the case of orthodox Jews not to touch the body but merely to cover it and remove it to the mortuary unless it can be collected very quickly. In the case of most progressive Jews, the body can be laid out in the normal way, but it is advisable to check with the family or rabbi first. However, to avoid contact with the body of the deceased, it is advisable for a non-Jewish nurse to use disposable gloves. Always, the requirement for dignity and perfection of the body is stressed and, unless there is a medico-legal requirement, permission may not be given for post-mortem examination. For most Jews, cremation is not acceptable. It should, perhaps, be mentioned that there are no last rites of any kind, but that orthodox Jews do not leave a body unattended.

In all forms of Judaism, the body is treated with great respect. It is not usually flaunted — there is a strong tradition of modesty. It is regarded as the 'vessel of divine creation', as an important part of the divine scheme of things, to be treasured, cared for and fed. As a result, any attempts to cure the body are always well received. It is an intrinsic part of Judaism to try to heal the sick and to tend them and cherish them. Those who devote their lives to these ends are amongst the most highly respected in Jewish thought, quite apart from being appreciated personally by those for whom they care.

This whole attitude — very positive to nursing and related care — makes it easy for nurses to give enormous assistance to their Jewish patients. The positive emotions are already there. All that is needed is some further awareness of particular aspects of Judaism, from the dietary laws (barely mentioned in this chapter but consisting basically of prohibitions on pork, most game, and shellfish, plus special requirements on slaughtering of meat (*shechitah*) and not mixing milk and meat) and festivals, to the Sabbath with all its significance, to the emphasis on study, to the life-affirming ethic of Judaism and to the value placed on the human body. All this is important. But most important of all is the conveying of that sense of loving care which is the embodiment of that first principle of Judaism '*pikkuach nefesh*' — 'The saving of life' — which is also the first principle of the nursing ethic of caring for patients, with love.

CHAPTER 8

THE HINDU PERSPECTIVE

Religion has an important place in the life of Hindu patients. Hinduism, one of the oldest religions in the world, 'constitutes a very complex but largely continuous whole, and since it covers the whole of life it has religious, social, economic, literary, and artistic aspects' (*New Encyclopedia Britannica* 1974). Individual Hindus differ in their religious beliefs, practices and values. Though Hindu society may appear to embody inconsistent varieties within itself, its bond of unity lies deep within its structure. To some, religion may consist of certain popular beliefs and rituals, whereas for others to be a Hindu is to be guided by a philosophy without any significant attachment to any form of ritualistic practices or worship. Even then, religion is a way of life to all and they have some things in common. For example, dietary habits, attitudes towards traditional or modern medicine, their hygienic practices of daily bathing, or placing importance on the opinions of pundits or senior family members in making decisions, for instance when surgery is advised. The code of Manu prescribed detailed rules for diet, personal hygiene and the routine of daily living.

At the onset it is necessary to have some basic understanding of the Hindu ethos and the beliefs which guide the Hindu community. The Hindu design for living suggests that man's life should be divided (Tagore 1962) into four parts:

1 *Brahmacharya*, the period of education.
2 *Gārhasthya*, that of the world's work.
3 *Vānapastha*, the retreat for the loosening of ties and worldly attachments.
4 *Pravrajyā* or *yati*, the awaiting of freedom through death.

Hindu sages did not merely stress learning from books in life's first stage, namely education, but they emphasized *brahmacharya* or disciplined living to strengthen character. After the period of education comes the period of worldly life when the individual fulfils his obligations and duties as a householder and citizen. It is believed that wisdom is not complete except through the full living of life, and at this stage one is expected to be actively involved in activities that promote the welfare of society and family.

The second stage of life having thus been spent, the decline of bodily powers is taken as a sign that it is approaching its natural end. In the third stage of life the individual, though aloof from the world, keeps in touch with it by giving the world his store of wisdom. Then comes the last stage when such relations are to be gradually severed and the spirit released to be united with the Supreme Being. Hindu sages thus never advised people to let life come to a sudden halt while work is in full swing, but to reach the stage of renunciation gracefully.

According to Hinduism, the fourfold purposes of life lie (Zimmer 1951) in the attainment of:

1 Material possessions or *Artha*.
2 Pleasure and love or *Kāma*.
3 Religious and material duties or *Dharma*.
4 Liberation from ignorance and world's general illusions or *Moksa*.

The ultimate reality of all true Hindus is directed towards the realization of *Moksa*, or the way to final emancipation. A sound body and a sound mind were regarded as prerequisites for this experience.

The Hindu religious text, the *Bhāgavadgītā*, presents three ways to salvation; the path of duties and discharge of social obligations, or *Karma-Mārga*; the path of knowledge, or the *Jhāna-Mārga*; and the path of devotion, or *Bhakti-Mārga* (*New Encyclopedia Brittanica* 1974). The regular practic of *Yoga* and the use of meditation is believed to help not only in maintaining bodily health, but also in improving mental health and peace of mind. For a Hindu, much significance is attached to the fulfilment of social duties following certain rituals and performing certain traditional rites for his family, group or caste. At the same time he attempts to formulate his own philosophy of life based upon his scriptures. This makes him both an individual as well as a social being with strong family ties.

A Hindu has a profound respect for life or *Ahimsa*. Thus, a vegetarian diet or particular food habits have become a way of life to many, though some vegetarians may not practise *Ahimsa* other than in their dietary habits.

The desire to maintain close and unbroken conduct with Nature and be one with animal and plant life has become inherent in the Hindu spirit.

Hindus generally accept the doctrine of rebirth. The doctrine of *Karma* teaches that all experience is the reward or punishment of previous actions. This being so, he believes that all that he faces in the world are the effects of his *Karma*. He knows that any misfortune or ill health he suffers is the reaction of his past *Karma*, either in this life or in his previous birth. This leads him to bear illness and diseases patiently in a spirit of acceptance. This helps one in accepting one's own condition calmly and also in developing tolerance, patience and forbearance during illness.

Some may mistakenly interpret such a doctrine as a fatalistic attitude towards life, but the philosophy of *Karma* encourages individuals in the pursuit of a better life through *Karma*. Health was often considered the reward of living by religious and moral laws.

Āyurveda, the science of life or the conception of Hindu medicine, is based on a well-defined philosophy which is shared equally by the patients and the physician. The routine of regular diet, sleep, defaecation, cleanliness of body and clothing, moderation in exercise and sexual practice are emphasized in *Āyurvedic* systems of medicine, which to this day remain the guiding principles of healthy living amongst the devout.

The caste system is one of the conspicuous characteristics of Hindu society. The rituals related to caste may not be overtly visible in many modern families, but are still a part of life for most. The importance given to caste varies among Hindu communities. On the basis of ritual purity, the Brahim groups occupied the highest place in Indian society, and the scheduled castes (or out castes) had the lowest status. However, in today's society social discrimination by caste is a punishable offence. Menstruating women and mourners are also considered as being untouchable because of ritual impurity. It is believed that low social status is the result of *Karma* in previous life, but by virtue of good and meritorious work in the present life may bring about a better position in the next.

Having given some insight into the background of Hindu patients, the spiritual needs and care of these patients in hospitals can be discussed in relation to patient care regimens and selected religious practices.

Bathing

A true Hindu believes in the purification of the body as a necessary step towards the purification of the mind and soul. For this, the Hindus give an importance to daily bathing in fresh water, preferably in running water such as a stream or river. A tub bath is not considered to be a satisfactory way of bathing because one comes out from the contaminated or unclean water in the tub. They believe that bathing not only makes a person feel physically clean but it also gives a feeling of spiritual well-being; for example, a bath is taken to mark the beginning of a new day and is always taken on auspicious occasions. A patient going for surgery may find a bath very important to begin his life that day. Although certain hours for bathing may not have special relevance, the usual preference is early in the morning, especially for elderly people. The washing of one's body as a part of the daily religious rite is common among devout Hindus. Ritual purity is considered as an approach to *dharma* (religious law). Bathing, the ceremonial use of water, and a variety of expiatory rites are just some of the means of purification. Some studies have also shown that a number of patients are happy to have their family help them bathe (e.g. McGorman 1971).

Food habits

Washing of hands and rinsing of the mouth before and after meals and cleanliness in the preparation and handling of food are important aspects of Hindu life. Many Hindus are vegetarian, and within a family the women are often more strict than the men in their dietary habits. Hindus do not eat beef or even eat other foods touched by it while cooking or serving, and they have strong feelings about this taboo. Some patients may like their food to be brought from home because they would not want to take food cooked by a member of a caste lower than theirs. A few patients may ask for home food because of religious reasons, but most of them may find hospital food unfamiliar and less appetizing. It would be necessary to give special permission to the former group for home food in deference to their religious belief and personal taste. The nurse is often required to explain the special dietary needs of a patient to the relatives, especially in relation to the use of oil and spices in cooking, so that the food which is brought from home is not harmful.

Foods may be considered to be stimulating and cooling and used according to one's state of health, the seasons and the weather. Hindus believe in 'hot' and 'cold' foods, although the basis of classifying foods in this way is not very clear. Many believe that there is a relationship between food and the seasons of the year, and it is quite likely that such fruits as oranges or plums would not be eaten in particular seasons even if they are plentiful, cheap and readily available.

Orthodox Hindu widows observe strict dietary rules, in that most are vegetarian and consider that such food items as meat, fish, eggs, onion, garlic, etc. cause excitement in a person.

It is important to remember that most Indians, irrespective of their religion, are sensitive to issues of food and diet. Anger, annoyance or anxiety are sometimes expressed through food, i.e. refusal to eat. However, food patterns vary from community to community, and often the dissatisfaction may arise from unfamiliarity. The nurse needs to find out whether dissatisfaction or unwillingness to accept the food is due to religious belief or not. Unfamiliarity or dislike of a particular method of cooking may be to blame. When asked to give dietary advice, especially to pregnant women, anaemic patients, and the mothers of infants, the nurse has to begin by finding out the dietary habits and practices of her Hindu patients.

Fasting

Fasting for religious purposes is most common among elderly, or widowed Hindu women. For special religious festivals, many men and women fast regularly on specific days of the week. For example, Tuesdays and Fridays are often observed as complete fast or semi-fast days in the north of India. Consequently, patients with diabetes mellitus, fluid and electrolyte imbalance or kidney disease may require a thorough explanation of the importance of dietary therapy, and the possible effects of long hours of fasting.

Grooming

Nudity is considered indecent, and therefore Hindu women may be reluctant to undress completely for medical examination. Privacy and adequate covering are very important, and an ankle-length gown which opens down the back should be available, especially when women are examined by a male doctor, but often an explanation will suffice. Hindu women often require sensitive and intelligent questioning to divulge their personal medical history, especially in respect of genitourinary problems.

The *Caraka Samhita* lays down an elaborate code regarding the duties and social status of physicians. According to the *Carak*, the physician must not attend a woman in the absence of her husband or guardian (Ray and Gupta 1965).

Certain items of jewellery are especially significant to Hindu married women, similar to the sacredness of the wedding ring for Christians. Similarly, some men wear the sacred thread around their bodies which carry religious and sentimental meaning for them. These should not be removed unless absolutely necessary and the person is willing to cooperate. A Bengali married woman wears an iron bangle around her left wrist, while married women from southern India and the province of Maharashtra wear a special chain and locket, and married and unmarried Sikh men and women wear a steel bangle around their right wrist. Therefore, care should be taken not to remove these inadvertently, and if necessary their removal must be explained in advance and the patient's cooperation obtained. Such jewellery may look like mere ornaments of decoration but they have sacred sentimental values attached to them, and their removal may affect the patient psychologically.

Privacy

Traditional Hindu women do not mix socially with unrelated men. Physical contact between men and women, even shaking hands, is generally discouraged socially, but touching and other tactile ways of expressing care and concern are appreciated, if the other member is not of the opposite sex. Hindu patients are also more relaxed in treatments requiring undressing, such as physiotherapy, where men and women are segregated in separate cubicles or rooms. In addition, Hindu women patients prefer female doctors for gynaecological or obstetric problems.

The role of visitors

Strong familiy ties often play a role in health and health care. The nurse should anticipate that many visitors will seek access to a Hindu patient. It is not only the relatives who will want to see the sick person, but the patient will like to see family around him. This is not usually allowed owing to the visiting policies of the hospital, but sometimes the rules should be relaxed for the social well-being of the patient. If the rules for restricted visiting are not strictly observed by friends and relatives, the nurse should be very understanding. She should listen to the points of view of the relatives and the patient and try to explain and interpret hospital regulations to them in terms of the patient's well-being.

Auspicious days and the wearing of charms

Some Hindus may look for an auspicious day, as decided by Pundits or family elders, to start a risky job or event. Such forecasting is often based on astrology. Therefore, it is necessary to appreciate why a Hindu patient may want to undergo surgery on a particular day, and why that day is considered more important than others. Also, some may wish to wear charms and amulets as lockets around their necks. Such beliefs should be respected even if the nurse may find them illogical and irrelevant, and charms should not be removed unless necessary or without explanation.

Worship

Most Hindus would like to have some time set aside for meditation and prayer, but it is not necessary to have a fixed time during the day. It is an individual practice. Early hours of the morning are often used by elderly men and women for prayer or reciting scriptures. Some may find it convenient to pray in bed or at the bedside, but some may prefer to have a quiet and clean room for worship. Some may like to keep under their pillow a small idol, or a picture of God, praying beads (like a rosary), or blessings (flowers, charms, etc.). Besides having religious connotations these provide a strong psychological support to the patient and help in his recovery. Hindus worship innumerable gods and goddesses. Some may worship one only, others many of the favourites (*ista devata*).

Hindu worship or *pūjā* is usually in image worship and consists of different stages. Normally individuals will perform these themseves, but on many occasions — such as festivals, auspicious days and marriages — they might employ a Brahmin officiant to help. Menstruating women and women in the postnatal period are considered unclean, and are not allowed to perform *pūjā*, touch the idol, or even enter the temple. There are many religious festivals, and divine assistance is implored on almost every occasion.

As in many other religions, the motives for observing religious practices may vary from a desire to please God to achieving the personal ultimate reality. Some Hindus, therefore, may be very particular about daily rituals of worship and prayer, while others may not. But there are innumerable ways of doing this. To many, religious practices are personal and do not always have to conform to group practices. To some, the acts of praying or performing rites may be most important, especially before starting every new day, new work, or undergoing surgery. There are others who strongly believe that right conduct can help in the preservation of physical and mental health. This makes it difficult to assess the spiritual needs of the Hindu patient, as religious practices are highly personalized.

Birth and death

Like any other human being, Hindus enjoy the birth of newborn in the family and grieve for a death.

Most of the rituals associated with birth and postnatal care are practised at home. These are mainly in terms of the mother's diet, and isolation of postnatal mothers and newborn from a few days to a few weeks; the period will vary in different Hindu communities. This is one way of giving much needed rest to the mother, as well as preventing contamination of mother and baby, and allowing her time to take care of a neonate. However, several reasons have now made such practices obsolete in urban areas; for example, shortage of space in overcrowded houses, inability to get home help, the nuclear family system, and non-availability of leave for working mothers.

Most Hindu mothers prefer to breastfeed their babies, and tend to be reluctant to start supplementary foods. In some communities they observe a religious ceremony (*annaprasan*) for introducing solid foods, usually cereals.

The nurse may often find the Hindu mother holding a dressed baby with a black mark (*tikka*) on the forehead. This is done to try to ward off evil. Such practices do not require any special nursing intervention, but call for a show of respect for the beliefs of others.

Death is often accepted philosophically by the dying person, as well as by the relatives. The religious outlook helps them to accept the inevitable; however, there are some rituals, which vary from place to place. In some communities, families prefer to place the dead body on the floor rather than the bed or cot, and some like oil lamps to be lit, and incense burnt near the dead. Cremation is the method of choice for disposal of the dead.

The *Srēda* ceremony is a death rite which is performed for the benefit of the deceased, when food offerings and other gifts are made to Brahims. As in many other religions, the Hindu priest performs certain religious rites after each death. The observation of a period of isolation or segregation after birth and death has a religious sanction.

Expression of grief has various forms. Some may cry loudly, hugging and embracing, and others may only show sadness in their faces. Touch is an important and meaningful act in expressing grief and sympathy, such as holding hands, touching shoulders, face or head, or even embracing. The overt expression of grief is not considered to be bad conduct; on the contrary, it is thought to be mentally healthy and to restore peace of mind.

Although the relatives may ask for special grooming or dressing of the deceased, there is usually no restriction among Hindus concerning the touching of the body by non-Hindus in the performance of care. However, if a post-mortem examination is to be performed, it will be necessary to talk to the relatives about it and to let them voice their concerns from both an ethical and religious point of view. There is, on the whole, a feeling of awe and respect for the dead body and many Hindus find the concept of post-mortem repugnant. This is often interpreted as showing a lack of respect for the departed.

Summary

While caring for a Hindu patient the nurse should remember that each patient is an individual who will be very different in his beliefs and values from other Hindus, whilst having some things in common. For example, the Hindu family is a closed unit, but the extended families living outside of India are mostly nuclear families who may not have the framework of support to which to turn in time of need. However, even in modern society, families care for their elderly members, providing a richness in the life of the elderly person, especially in the traditional Hindu homes of rural India. Taking care of elderly family members was traditionally thought to be a way of earning merit for performing obligation, and accumulating good religious deed to one's credit.

Often it is claimed that there exists in the mind of the orthodox Hindu a belief that illness is due to a spell cast upon him by an enemy, or to an act of God, or other supernatural power. Although this does not go with the rationale of modern medicine, to condemn it or ignore it disrespectfully may lead to rejection or distrust in the patient which could be detrimental to his welfare. As Wilcocks (1965) claimed, 'It is a good rule not to treat people as inferiors, whoever they are. In the end, we hope, example will do the convincing for us'.

Some Hindu practices appear to have generated from or into superstitious beliefs but, as with many other religions, underlying these there are many practical, social and logical justifications connected with spiritual upliftment, or a desire for a whole and meaningful life. Spiritual needs are more self- or family orientated than community based, and Hindus have various ways of worshipping. What one sees generally, and on the surface, are more akin to religious folk practices than true religious practices. Nevertheless, such folk practices also have implications for the planning and giving of care. Because human beings are constantly reacting to their environment, family traditions and social and religious expectations, it is important to find out the patient's attitude as to what will or will not be acceptable, and to try to accommodate the patient's view or habits within the care plan. Hence, it is important to identify these needs and care for the whole person, especially as Hindus hold such individual beliefs and attitudes.

The concepts of health and disease prevalent among Hindus today are a mixture of all that has been known in India from the earliest times to the era of modern medicine. But, throughout the ages, Hindus have emphasized the spiritual perspective in the maintenance of health. Optimum health for spiritual attainment is a goal cherished and highly valued by devout Hindus.

References

McGorman, M N (1971) A Study of Spiritual Needs of Hindu Patients in Hospital, Master of Nursing Thesis, University of Delhi

New Encyclopedia Britannica (1974) Macropedia, Volume 8, page 888, Encyclopedia Britannica

Ray, P and Gupta, H N (1965) Caraka Samhitā (A Scientific Synopsis), National Institute of Sciences in India

Wilcocks, C (1965) Medical Advance; Public Health and Social Evolution, Pergamon Press

Tagore, R (1962) The Universal Man, Asia Publishing House

Zimmer, H (1951) Philosophies of India, in J Campbell (Editor) Pantheon Books

Further reading

Hartig, E E (1954) Health and Medicine in India, Master of Arts Thesis, The Kennedy School of Missions of the Hartford Seminary Foundations

Henley, A (1980) Practical care of Asian patients, Nursing, 16: 683–686

Jolly, J (1951) Indian Medicine, translated from German and supplemented with notes by G G Kashikar, 196/27 Sadashiv, Poona-2, India

CHAPTER 9

THE MUSLIM PERSPECTIVE

The origins and philosophies of Islam

'Whether or not history will stress the technical achievements of this age, more or less than its efforts to understand human nature, the guidance beliefs of people are products of their moral imagination' (Henderson 1978). Many books, journal articles and other learning media can be cited to stress the importance of understanding the nature of human beings. Religious beliefs, ethical concepts, moral values, or the meaning of life lie at the roots of each individual, and the achievement of health is, to some extent, dependent on harmony between belief and behaviour.

There are many religions being practised in the world today and prominent among them is Islam. The word Islam means 'peaceful submission to God's will'. The term can refer to the faith of muslim which is based on the teaching of Muhammad (or Mohammed), as recorded in the Qur'ān (or Koran). Islam can also refer to the whole body of Muslims (or Moslems), their civilization and the countries in which their religion is dominant.

Islam is the most recent of the great living religions. Its founder, Muhammad, is said to have been born in Mecca, in present-day Saudi Arabia, in AD 570. He grew up in the religions tradition of his community, but he is said to have been disturbed by its polytheism, its immorality at religious gatherings, its intertribal anarchy and the bloodshed of ensuing wars. When he was about 40 years of age, he went to a cave at the base of Mount Hira, near Mecca, to brood over the change in his religious beliefs. One night, known as the Night of Power and Excellence, the vision of an angel appeared to him, and as the Messenger of God, spoke to him, 'In the name of thy Lord, who created Man of a blood clot ... Thy Lord is the Most Generous who taught not by the pen, taught Man what he knew not ...'. (Arberry 1955). Although beset by doubts after this meeting with the Angel Gabriel, he assumed the role of prophet, reciting in verse the revelations of the Lord (or Allah). His followers wrote down these sayings which eventually formed the Qur'ān. These sayings can be organized under the following headings.

Iman, or articles of faith

A belief in God, or Allah, who stands alone and who is the most powerful and merciful, and who — on the day of judgement — will save believers and place them in paradise.

Ihsan, or right conduct

Such conduct includes believing in God, in the Last Day, the Angels, the Book (Qur'ān), and the Prophets. It includes giving to kinsmen, orphans, the needy, travellers, beggars and the ransoming of slaves. Good conduct also includes praying, the giving of alms, fulfilling covenants, enduring with fortitude any misfortune, hardship or peril, being kind to one's parents, and the elderly, never exchanging what is good for the corrupt, and avoiding fornication. Good conduct includes marriage; 'marrying women as seems good to you, two, three or four: but if you fear you will not be equitable then only one'. Right conduct includes dietary laws, for example the blood and flesh of swine and carrion are prohibited. Gambling is also prohibited, as are the use of divining rods, worship of idols, taking of alcohol, etc.

Ibadat, or religious duty

This is based on the 'Five Pillars' (Al-Arkan).

1. Repetition of the Creed (Shahada). 'La ilāha, illa Allāh; Muhammad rasūl Allāh' (There are no Gods but Allah, and Muhammad is the Prophet of Allah).

2. Prayer *(Salat)* five times each day. These prayers take place at dawn, noon, mid-afternoon, sunset and the fall of darkness. The devout bow low towards Mecca.
3. Almsgiving *(Zakāt).* This is now mostly voluntary.
4. Fasting during the sacred month of Ramadan. No food is taken from the time when a white thread can be distinguished from a black at dawn, until sundown, when the difference is no longer perceptible to the eye.
5. Pilgrimage (Hajj). Once during the lifetime a pilgrimage is made to Mecca during the sacred month of *Dhu-al-Hajji.* Pilgrims join the sacred circumambulation at the Kaaba at Mecca, the Lesser and Greater Pilgrimages, and the Great Feast.

When Muhammad began his teaching he established himself in the city known now as Medina, where he built a Mosque and introduced services on Fridays in the same way that Christians recognize Sundays and Jews worship on Saturdays. In AD 630 he conquered Mecca by force of arms and tried to unify the various factions in Arabia under Islam, but died in AD 632 before this could be accomplished. His principle aim was to teach people how to behave, and what to do in order to pass the reckoning on the Day of Judgement. That is why Islamic law is a particular system of duties, comprising ritual, legal and moral obligations on the same footing, and bringing them all under the authority of the same religious command.

The Qur'ān places equal emphasis on the physical and the transcendental yearning of Man and seeks to harmonize them. Thus it lays down for humanity a comprehensive ideal, which consists of the cultivation of five achievements:

1. Holiness, based on a dynamic, vibrant and living Faith in God, an earnest and courageous pursuit of the Truth, and an ever-present consciousness of Final Accountability.
2. A sound and comprehensive Morality.
3. Social, economic and political Justice.
4. Knowledge, in all its dimensions.
5. Aesthetic Grace.

Achievement of all of these will result in the conquest of harmful propensities within the individual and the physical environment, or Nature. The watchwords in the pursuit of the Ideal are: Holiness, Love for Humanity, Truth, Justice, Beauty (of mind), Discipline and Progress; while the concept of Unity permeates the entire movement towards the

Ideal, and the motto 'simple living, hard labour, and high thinking' forms the wheel of progress (Ansari 1975).

Therefore, it can be claimed that the Islamic concept of illness is based on Man's inability to harmonize himself as a physical and spiritual being within this environment.

The Islamic calendar and religious festivals

The Islamic calendar is a lunar reckoning from the year of the hegira, the year when Muhammed moved from Medina to Mecca. It runs in cycles of 30 years, of which 11 are designated leap years of 355 days instead of the common 354 days. The extra day is added to the last month of the year, called *Dhu-al-Hajji*. The other months consist alternately of 30 and 29 days each, and a month begins at sunset. The commencement of any month is not fixed or static but fluctuates from year to year. For example, Muharram (New Year) may begin on December 23rd or January 3rd, while Ramadan may commence on various dates in August. *Dhu-al-Hajji*, the time of pilgrimage, usually begins in middle or late November (*World Almanac Book of Facts* 1976).

The main religious festivals in the Islamic year, although they may be differently observed by the various divisions within Islam, are as follows. There are two feast days:

1. *Id al-Fitr*, or 'little feast', which takes place on the first day of the month of *Shawwal* (about September).
2. *Id al-Adha*, or the 'Great Feast', which takes place on the tenth day of the month of *Dhu-al-Hajji* (about November). This feast represents the ritual offering of allowed animals, when pilgrims to Mecca have returned half-way from their Great Pilgrimage.

There are three main Islamic festivals:

1. *Muharran*, or New Year, which is observed on the first day of the first month. It is observed by the Shi'ites with lamentation associated with the death of the prophet Ali and his sons.
2. *Mawli an-Nabi*, the festival of the Prophet's birthday. This takes place on the twelfth day of the month of *Rabi Al-Awwal* (about Easter).
3. *Lailat al-Mir'aj*, or the festival of the Prophet's Night Journey. This is usually observed on the night before the twenty-seventh day of the

month of *Rajab* (June), when the Mosques and particularly the minarets are illuminated, and accounts of the Journey are read.

Some implications for health and nursing care

Having offered some insight into the origins and philosophies of the Islamic religion, the spiritual needs and care of patients in hospital can now be discussed in respect of the patient's care regimen and selected religious practices.

Bathing

Bathing is an important aspect of the Islamic religion, more especially if it takes the form of purification. Before attending Friday prayers it is considered preferable to bathe within an hour of the ceremony, so the ablution is performed for purification of the mind as well as the body. Ritual purity is considered as an approach to 'religious law'. Beauty, as an ideal of Qur'ānic philosophy, commits the pursuer to gracefulness and beautification in every aspect of life. Cleanliness, therefore, becomes the watchword in respect of all actions involving the body, dress and the environment (Ansari 1975).

Therefore, it is important that the nurse helps the patient perform these ritual purifications, or where necessary the relative should be allowed to do so. Because of the importance of bathing, the body is washed even after death. The hands of the dead patient are then placed as in prayer, i.e. descending parallel to the body, the corpse is enshrouded and is buried without a coffin. Before the head of the body is covered over, the relatives may say farewell, and the imam, or Islamic minister, may recite some verses from the Qur'ān.

Food habits and taboos

Washing of hands before and after meals, as well as rinsing out the mouth, are important in the life of a devout Muslim. This, however, may be more cultural than religious. Many (but not all) Muslims are vegetarians. It states in the Qur'ān (chapter 11, verse 87) that, 'Forbidden unto you [for food] are carrion, and blood, and swineflesh, and that over which is invoked the name of other than Allah, and the strangled, the felled [i.e. killed by a blow], and the dead through falling from a height, and that which hath been killed by horns, and that which hath been [partly] eaten by wild beasts — saving that which ye make lawful [death by a stroke or slash], and that which hath been slaughtered on the altars'. The Qur'ān also states, 'And eat not that whereon Allah's name has not been mentioned, for lo, it is an abomination'.

Consequently, Muslims have a very strong feeling about the type of food they eat, and some patients may want to have their food brought in from home. It would be necessary to seek special permission for a Muslim patient to take food in difference to his religious beliefs. If the food is to be brought from home, adequate explanation must be offered to the family in respect of what is allowed, and extra effort must be made when explaining a special diet to the Muslim patient. People are sensitive to diet irrespective of their religious beliefs, and because food patterns vary from community to community, dissatisfaction may often arise simply because of unfamiliarity. The nurse should take steps to enquire about the reason for a Muslim patient refusing food. However, when a Muslim finds himself in a country dominated by different cultural and religious habits, he is allowed to eat their food, so long as it is not one of the foods previously mentioned. The Qur'ān states, 'This day are (all) good things made lawful for you. The food of those who have received the Scripture is lawful for you (provided it consists of lawful things), and your food is lawful for them'.

Fasting during the month of Ramadan is compulsory to every Muslim, man or woman, who has reached the age of puberty, and who is physically and mentally sound. No food or drink should be taken from dawn to dusk each day, as described earlier in this chapter. However, when a person is ill, either in hospital or at home, and when it is absolutely necessary to his health, such a person may eat and drink during the prohibited hours. Treatment is seen as necessary to sustain life, in order to fulfill life obligations. It becomes necessary for patients with certain diseases or illnesses — e.g. diabetes mellitus, fluid and electrolyte imbalance, or renal disease — to be told the importance of dietary therapy and the possible effects of long hours of fasting. When the patient is well enough he or she will fast for the period of time lost through illness.

Privacy

Islam strongly restricts social interaction between physically mature men and women, more especially if they are unrelated. However, touching and other interactions are permitted if the toucher is not of the opposite sex. Therefore, Muslim patients who require a medical examination may feel more relaxed when men and women are segregated in separate rooms. When exposure is necessary, women patients prefer female doctors. This strong belief is held within all Muslim society and should be respected both by medical and by nursing staff. When a female nurse or physician is not available and the female patient needs immediate attention then it is permitted for the opposite sex to take action, for Allah is 'oft-forgiving, and most merciful'.

Worship

'Thy Lord has decreed that ye worship none but Him'. The Holy Qur'ān demands not merely formal obedience, but obedience with all one's heart. Not only obedience but total surrender, with indivisible loyalty to God. Indeed, a Muslim's attitude to God should be that of worship, in which his role is that of total humility, and remembrance of God should be constant. The Qur'ān stresses that the wise are, 'those who remember Allah standing, sitting, and reclining', because, 'Lo, in the remembrance of Allah hearts do find serene tranquility and steady peace'.

Islam stresses the importance of regular prayers for the remembrance of Allah. These regular or obligatory prayers should be performed punctually at the appointed times, five times each day as described earlier. Because of the importance of these prayers, no other person is involved. Even when the patient is bedridden, or is paralysed, no one can perform these prayers on his behalf. Here the nurse has a duty of either bringing the opportunity for prayer to the patient — by screening the bed and providing clean sheets and water — or by taking the patient to a service.

When articles for use in prayer are brought from home, the nurse should respect them and, if consistent with the welfare of other patients, allow patients to keep such articles with them, or nearby. The early hours of the morning are often used by elderly Muslim men and women for prayer and reciting scriptures. Patients may be happy to pray on the bed, or at the bedside; others may prefer a quiet and clean room for prayer. As well as maintaining religious obligations prayers may provide strong psychological support in the recovery process.

Because the motives for observing religious practices are a desire to please God, and to achieving the ultimate reality, some Muslims may be very particular about the daily rituals of worship, while others may not. To most people religious practices are personal and do not always conform to group practices. Such personalized practices may make it difficult to assess the needs of each individual Muslim patient. Nevertheless, a nurse should try to learn how religion, ritual and values affect the meaning of illness, the concept of therapy, and hence the treatment which the patient may be willing to undergo.

Summary and concluding comments

The ideal of promotion of life, in accordance with Qur'ānic philosophy, rests in the effort for establishing sound physical, moral and mental or spiritual health. The duties that emerge in respect of physical health include avoiding unhealthy food and drink and refraining from gluttony, taking all nutrients in balanced quantities and indulging in recurrent fasting besides the obligatory fast of Ramadan. Muslims should indulge in healthy exercise including sport and ensure proper rest. For moral health, Muslims must maintain purity of conscience and engage in effort for achieving sound moral behaviour in their communities. For mental or spiritual health the Muslim must try to cultivate a living and dynamic relationship with God — to perform the minimum basic obligatory prayers, to fast during Ramadan, to give a fixed portion of one's surplus wealth for the benefit of others — solely for the love of God. The Muslim must seek to avoid any superstition or other hindrance to his devotion to God.

However, man should not be considered as a composite of several levels such as body, mind, or soul, but rather as a multidimensional unity. The extent to which people believe that health is dependent on peace of mind, or emotional balance, determines their willingness to assign to the imam or priest a place in health institutions and agencies. Since nurses are with patients more than ·any other health workers, they have the greatest opportunity to listen and to be the patient's confidante. The more spirituality nurses have, the more comfortable they will be in discussing spiritual questions, and the more likely it will be that people, whether patients or their families, will confide in them. Consequently, nurses should listen with interest to anything which patients or relatives say about their ethical values, spiritual needs, or religious beliefs, noting any aspect of care or treatment which runs counter to these values or makes it impossible for the patient to act consistently with his or her religious beliefs.

When a Muslim patient expresses a wish to see a spiritual advisor the nurse should communicate this need to an appropriate person. However, she can also read prayers or some religious literature to the Muslim patient if it is requested by him or his family.

Finally, the knowledge which the nurse has of religion, and her ability to serve people of any faith with understanding, determines the range and quality of her usefulness. Men and women in nursing, who have honestly faced the serious questions of life, will be more effective and more comfortable in their giving than those who have not, even when they work with people in a crisis.

References

Ansari, M F (1975) The Qur'ānic Foundations and Structure of Muslim Society, Industrial Education Foundation

Arberry, A T (1955) The Qur'ān Interpreted, George Allen & Unwin

Henderson, V (1978) Principles and Practice of Nursing, Macmillan

World Almanac Book of Facts (1976) page 498, Newspaper Enterprise Association

PART THREE

SPIRITUAL CARE IN NURSING

CHAPTER 10

SPIRITUAL CARE IN ACUTE ILLNESS

Introduction

In the past, when hospitals in Europe were religious institutions, the problem of spiritual care did not arise. A united Christian principle underlay patient care, and all were perpetually aware of their responsibility in respecting the supernatural property of human life. Today, secularization has permeated institutional care and has resulted in the designation of a low priority to all spiritual matters. Also, society's advancement in technology has altered the nature of nursing. Machines have taken over tasks nurses once performed, methods have become highly technical, and specialties have replaced the general wards of yesterday. The result has been an intense interest in the intricacies of medical science and, unfortunately, a tendency to accord priority to the disease rather than the person.

In nursing, it has been easy, particularly in high-technology acute areas, to forget that caring is, 'concern for the totality of the recipient of nursing' (Lewis 1976), that is, concern for the body, mind and soul. The mechanistic, technical aspect of care has been amplified at the expense of that unique quality of care which consists in perceiving and meeting all the needs of the patient.

A depersonalized approach is particularly likely in an Intensive Care unit, which has come to represent the technological élite of the nursing profession. Dame Catherine Hall, addressing an International Intensive Care Conference in London, in 1982, commented on the aim of the British course in intensive care nursing, organized by the National Board of the UKCC whose general aim is to train the nurse, 'in order to be fully competent to meet not only the specialized technical needs of the patient, but also the emotional and mental stresses of patients, relatives and staff'. Dame Catherine stated that, 'This aim recognises that, whilst technology plays an important part in intensive care nursing, the nurse must always be concerned with the patient as a whole person, with his need for total care — physical, social and ... spiritual'.

The vast majority of nurses caring for the acutely ill are familiar with the need-centred theory of nursing. Physical and, increasingly, psychological, and social needs are given attention. Why then, is no united effort made to ensure that spiritual needs are met consistently? Why is a large part of spiritual care left to the discretion and conscience of individual nurses? In many ways, spiritual care is subjective, and its success rests upon the meaning of conversations between individual patients and nurses. It depends on the degree of trust and understanding exhibited, and on the extent to which the nurse can, from her experience, actively reinforce the patient's belief and help alleviate his fears.

Obviously, if nurses aspire to give consistent spiritual care, the problems inherent in such an intuitive approach are numerous. First, briefly, it is unreasonable in a pluralist society to expect complete understanding between each nurse and patient. Nurses usually find difficulty in giving spiritual comfort to patients whose beliefs and values differ radically from their own. Secondly, nurses vary greatly in their spiritual awareness. Some have always been concerned in detecting spiritual needs, whilst many others lack confidence in this area. Thirdly, the role of the nurse in relation to that of the chaplain is as yet ill defined. Finally, regardless of the professional expectations of the nurse in spiritual care, in caring for the acutely ill nurses are undoubtedly frequently confronted with deep spiritual problems, such as fear of death. The lack of personal and emotional preparation of nurses for this task should be evident to all in the profession.

The aim of this chapter, therefore, is to examine different aspects and levels of spiritual care in acute illness, beginning with a brief definition of the spirit and spiritual needs, and followed by a study on intensified spiritual need in acute illness. Finally, a number of practical, organizational aspects of spiritual care will be discussed and different levels of care suggested.

Spiritual needs

Spiritual needs, indeed the spirit itself, are difficult to define, because of the different meanings which the terms connote to persons of varying religions and sects. For the purposes of this chapter, four fundamental spiritual needs have been chosen because of their applicability in the critical stages of acute illness. The nature of these needs is based on the premise that the human personality is predisposed to a relationship with a Supernatural Being. Although it is not within the scope of such a short study to pursue solutions to the problems posed by these needs, what will be said makes the assumption that the ultimate fulfilment of man's spiritual need may only be found when he enters into a faith relationship with his God.

Meaning

Human beings always pursue meaning; they seek reasons to explain the experiences which they undergo throughout the course of life. The humanist explains his experiences in totally secular terms and ceases to have meaning at the horizon of the human view, whilst the religious believer looks to the 'beyond', and recognizes human meaning in a wider context of eternal meaning. The latter is aware of his need for a relationship with God and derives meaning from that relationship.

Love

The human spiritual need for love is universal. It includes both the need to love and to be loved. Maslow, in his hierarchy of human needs, described it as a sense of belonging. Lewis (1971) drew a distinction between two loves — what he called 'need-love' and 'gift-love'. In ordinary human relationships, he claimed, 'need-love' always predominates. 'Gift-love', by contrast, is much rarer; it is selfless, gracious and undemanding, and human relationships rarely contain it. Lewis believes that man's love for God must always be a 'need-love', whilst God's love for man is the epitome of 'gift-love'. The relationship between God and man, therefore, is such that man loves God because he needs the 'gift-love' which God affords.

Self-worth

The third fundamental spiritual need of man is to be aware that he possesses value in himself. Maslow has claimed that all people in society, with a few pathological exceptions, have a need or desire for a stable, firmly based, usually high evaluation of themselves; in other words, for self-respect, and for the esteem of others. It is questionable, however, whether social and psychological fulfilment suffice in satisfying such 'esteem' needs. Everyone needs some spiritual or moral basis for his idea of self-worth. Such needs may be met by an awareness that one has value before one's God, and within the universe. The Christian response goes further and teaches that an individual may have a relationship with God, and may be integrated in doing so, into a community of faith, i.e. the church.

Hope

Everyone needs something to hope for in the future. Life would be extremely depressing if nothing but gloom lay ahead. The non-believer's hope ceases at the end of mortal life, while the believer's hope is an eternal one, transcending the barriers of death. The need of the believer, therefore, during acute illness, is for assurance and reinforcement of the belief which sustains his hope.

Spiritual needs in acute illness

The spiritual needs of an individual are intensified when he is acutely ill in hospital, not least by his search for meaning in suffering and death. Other factors include vulnerability in an impersonal, mechanistic environment, coupled with separation from religious ritual, which may have been a crucial instrument in the growth of an individual's faith.

A number of situations seem to precipitate a particular need for renewal of meaning and comfort in faith.

The threat of imminent death

It is difficult to ascertain the feelings of someone when they find themselves in a life-threatening situation, since individual responses are so different. Kubler-Ross (1969) claimed that fear is one universal human response, along with denial, isolation, anger and depression. She wrote that, 'Death is a fearful, frightening happening, and the fear of death is universal, even if we think we have mastered it on many levels'.

The needs of a person facing death span many areas, none more critical than the spiritual. The need for meaning is rarely stronger than when an acutely ill patient witnesses the death of others and anticipates his own death. For those without a religious belief, death may create an area of meaninglessness and futility. Autton (1980) claimed that, 'Illness and the threat of death forces man to make sense of his experience in the world. Until he can place his experience in a framework of meaning, he is restless and uneasy. Anxiety, doubt, bitterness, frustrate his restoration to health'.

In order to explain beyond the horizon of death, most people turn to some kind of religion. The essence of religion gives a meaning to death which implies that biological death is not the end and, in this way, gives purpose to suffering and death, and hope for the life to follow.

When a person finds himself isolated in a strange, mechanistic environment, suffering pain and facing the possibility of death, the need to receive love is intensified. Many people rely heavily on family and friends, and perhaps hospital staff, for fulfilment of this need. Religious believers, whilst also needing and appreciating the love of close ones, depend ultimately on the love of their God, which for them surpasses any love a human being can offer and endures through and beyond death.

The need for self-worth sometimes changes nature when mortal life is in danger. Those who, in health, were concerned with the spiritual dimension of self-worth, i.e. spiritual worth before God, will tend to mature in that vein. On the other hand, those whose predominant need in health was worth before other human beings often change when acute illness strikes, and the threat of imminent death becomes realized. For the Christian, there is now a much stronger impetus to be worthy before God, since He alone has power through death. Hence the desire for all men to 'make peace with God' at the close of life.

Finally, hope is a vital component in the outlook of anyone facing death. The hope of the religious believer incorporates aspirations for the after-life. When awareness of one's mortality is stimulated, as in acute illness, anxiety often prevails, latent doubts are experienced and hope beyond death is sought.

Pain and suffering

A definition of pain is not easily made. Individual responses differ widely, and the subjective nature of pain makes objective assessment virtually impossible. The physical, psychological and social factors involved in pain responses are debatable, but on one or all of these levels the ability to cope with a particular kind of pain may undoubtedly vary from one person to another. For example, what produces anxiety and fear in one person may produce resilience and strength in another. In a situation where pain is not controlled, staying with a patient and attempting to share his experience would be supportive.

On a spiritual level, the religious beliefs of an individual may assist him in coping with pain, while the absence of such beliefs in another may intensify feelings of anxiety. The personal faith of individuals may also encourage them either to seek deliverance from pain or, on the contrary, to consider pain as a revelatory experience. That is to say, that the suffering entailed in their experience may strengthen their faith, and thus bring them closer to their God. In another sense, as Lewis (1971) claimed, pain is an instrument. It may create in a person an awareness of his need for a personal faith since, by suffering, he is brought closer to a recognition of evil in the world. Lewis wrote that, 'Until the evil man finds evil present in his existence, in the form of pain, he is enclosed in an illusion. Once pain has aroused him, he knows he is up against the real universe: he either rebels or makes some attempt at adjustment which, if pursued, will lead him to religion'.

The need to find meaning in suffering is problematic for the non-believer and believer alike. The non-believer has a natural framework within which to make sense of his painful situation, whilst the believer must accept that he is not immune from experiencing pain and must also resolve apparent contradictions between suffering and a God portrayed as a God of Love. In some types of acute illness, pain may result in an intensified search for meaning, whilst in others it may not. For example, acute appendicitis tends to cause excruciating pain, but the condition is easily operable and rarely provokes an individual to seek a spiritual meaning behind his suffering. On the other hand, the characteristic crushing pain of a myocardial infarction will often stir the individual to ask the question, 'Why me?' In a similar way the innocent victim of a road accident will inevitably search for meaning to an inexplicable occurrence.

The patient in pain experiences a certain vulnerability and dependency, as the relief of his symptoms depends on the standard of care administered by nursing staff. Not surprisingly, the patient is often in a state of irritability and tension; a state which might provoke an uncaring response from the nurse. It is at this time that the patient needs to receive unconditional, undemanding 'gift-love', from his God.

Indignity and embarrassment

Dignity is defined in *Collins English Dictionary* as, 'the state or quality of being worthy of honour'. It is closely related to the fulfilment of a person's need for self-worth. An individual to whom dignity has been accorded will feel that he is, in some way, worthy or important to someone. The religious view is that the spirit, being that aspect of man which is made in the image of God, gives man his dignity. This being the case, a nurse who looks upon her patients as individual human beings, each containing a unique spirit within him, can do little else but give them dignity.

Conversely, what produces indignity at a time of acute illness is a non-spiritual concern for the survival of the body, concentration on diseases rather than persons, and a cold, mechanistic preoccupation with the technical aspects of care. This type of attitude, sad to say, is particularly likely to prevail in high-powered intensive care units, where there is a strong tendency to look upon patients as challenges to science as opposed to human beings in need of personal care.

Embarrassment is not synonymous with indignity, although the two are related. Embarrassment is, by definition, 'a feeling of confusion or self-consciousness'. On certain occasions the emotion may be mild, and often pleasant, as every 'blushing bride' will recall. Embarrassment which introduces an acute sense of mortification, which is neither mild nor pleasant, can result from the introduction of a sudden state of dependency. This state is worsened when caring individuals are insensitive to the patient's need to remain as independent as possible under the circumstances. The spiritual need for self-worth is particularly significant in such situations, since a person who loses control of his body must feel, in a sense, that he is no longer worthy as a useful, independent, and dignified human being. It is then that a much deeper desire for worthiness before his God may assume full significance.

Spiritual care in acute illness

In health, spiritual needs are satisfied when a person outworks his faith in a way which is purposeful for him. During a period of acute illness, fresh challenges arise, and renewed meaning in faith is often sought. Furthermore, an individual, at such a time, may for many reasons find difficulty in understanding and preserving the implications of his faith without aid. The role of the nurse assumes great importance in this situation. Opportunity must be given for the patient to imbibe the meaning of his religion in a way which gives him fullest satisfaction. Every effort must be made to ensure that his worries reach a sympathetic ear, and that the best person is available to answer his questions.

When considering the practical aspects of spiritual care in acute illness, two points must be made at the outset. First, the implications of organizing care around task allocation are significant. If nurses do not have clearly defined motives behind their actions, and if they do not view the patient as a complete entity, then within a system of task allocation it is likely that spiritual care will be relegated to a very low priority level. Tasks that are overtly physical, and in some areas often technical, will be given top priority, and the more covert needs of a spiritual nature will tend to be ignored. The only feasible way of giving care which meets perceived spiritual need is through individualizing care by means of patient allocation. Under such a system of organization the patient is more likely to be seen comprehensively, that is with conglomerate needs of body, mind and soul. A deeper, more secure nurse–patient relationship is required if disclosure of personal spiritual worries is to take place.

The second point that should be emphasized is that the nurse and patient are two independent variables, each of whom differs from the other, in matters of faith, spiritual awareness and maturity. Consequently, it is necessary to set aside the ideal that every relationship will have the quality of a deep spiritual understanding. The analogy of a pyramidal structure of practice may be a useful way of introducing a discussion about ways in which nurses can care to the limits of their own abilities. The broad base of the pyramid can be taken to represent aspects of religious practice which every nurse, regardless of her beliefs, should be able to facilitate. Ascending the pyramid, a second level represents a deeper personal involvement between nurse and patient. Conversations at this level may, or may not, verge on the spiritual; and nurses, through their care and concern, often help patients resolve spiritual problems in an indirect way. At the apex of the pyramid a third, deep level of spiritual communion is seen, usually between a nurse and patient who share similar beliefs and values. At this level, the nurse is in a special position to administer to her patient fully, help to reinforce his faith, and assist him in meeting personal spiritual needs.

Religious practice

For many people, religious ritual is a very important component of faith, and of a normal lifestyle. Concerning Christianity, Lewis (1982) believed that, '...daily prayers and religious readings and church-going are necessary. We have to be continually reminded of what we believe. Neither this belief nor any other will automatically remain alive in the mind. It must be fed'. If acute illness and hospitalization suddenly prevent a person carrying out these practices then faith may wane, and spiritual problems arise. This is especially so in situations where the patient is in isolation for reasons of contagion, either to himself or others. Nursing staff in acute areas have an immense responsibility in helping such patients maintain rituals important to their faith. Barrier nursing is not a 'barrier' to the patient receiving the sacraments of his faith, unless the health care staff make it so.

There are a number of ways in which the nurse can give assistance. A bedside radio or television should be available, to enable patients to listen to religious broadcasts, particularly Sunday services. Alternatively, a tape recorder might be used, to play cassettes of services of the patient's particular faith, his own local church or chapel. Those who are fearful, anxious, depressed, debilitated, or simply lonely enjoy being reminded of religious practice at home. Many find that personal prayer is easier in an atmosphere of worship, than against a background of hurried activity and noises from machines. The mechanically ventilated patient in the intensive care unit who is known to be a religious believer may also derive comfort from sounds of worship, or religious music, although it is often impossible to ascertain the precise level of the patient's comprehension in such a situation. It is worth attempting, however, in the assumption that even in an unconscious patient a certain amount of sensory input can be imbibed. One should always precede such interventions with an explanation, in case the patient misconstrues the motive, and forms the idea that he is going to die.

A number of patients, even during a period of acute illness, are able to continue to read religious literature independently, while others may have to depend on the nurse to read to them. For example, a patient who has been drained of physical energy as a result of pain, anaesthesia, electrolyte imbalance, or a number of other factors, often finds it difficult to concentrate on reading, and may delight in having favourite passages from the Bible, or other texts, read aloud by the nurse, or a volunteer.

It is important to ensure privacy when the patient is praying, when his minister is visiting, or when sacraments are being received. This can be difficult, since many acute wards are centres of great activity. Constant noises and interruptions arise from the daily work of doctors, nurses, physiotherapists, technicians, cleaners, etc. — all necessarily demanding attention in respect of the patient situation. Sensitivity and discretion on the part of the nurse, along with the use of screens, should alleviate the problem to a large extent. Complete privacy in an intensive care unit, or accident and emergency department, is very difficult to achieve. A 'special' nurse may have to remain at the patient's side while sacraments are offered. Discretionary silence will help considerably, and a number of chaplains would invite the nurse, if she shares the patient's beliefs, to join in prayer.

Religion for many people is more than a personal faith; rather it is a way of life. Cultural restrictions concerning food, recreation, modesty, etc., are essential components of religious practices for many groups; for example, Jews, Hindus, Sikhs and Muslims. A nurse who albeit unwittingly neglects to respect these practices can offend her patient and cause him unnecessary anxiety. For example, an Asian woman, admitted to hospital as a surgical emergency, who has never been examined by a male doctor before will be understandably distressed at being stripped of clothing for a medical examination by the house medical officer on call. A nurse with understanding and knowledge of Asiatic religious practice could prevent distress occurring by either arranging for the patient to be cared for by female doctors and nurses, or, during the examination, ensuring that the woman is only undressed as much as necessary. It is worth pointing out that the caring nurse should see that any patient, especially a woman, is not unnecessarily exposed during examination, or treatment. The Asian woman may feel more comfortable if her husband is present, or gives her his permission for the examination to take place.

Whilst it is, perhaps, impossible for nurses to have an in-depth knowledge of all world religions, and their offshoots, there is no doubt that information on the mainstream religions, when stored on a ward, can enhance the delivery of total patient care. The problem of caring for the spiritual needs of religious minority groups, in any country, may be partly solved by careful assessment on admission. Simply writing in the nursing card index, 'Seventh Day Adventist', or 'Shi'ite Muslim', is not enough. When relatives or friends of the patient, or the patient himself, are not able to give details of the cultural restrictions imbibed in such religions the nurse should have source material readily at hand.

Personal spiritual care

From a nursing point of view, spiritual care would be relatively straightforward if it were confined to religious practice. There is a certain security in formality. However, spiritual activity can never be restricted to mere religious practice, nor can spiritual need be fulfilled successfully in a scientific, planned way. An expression of deep-rooted anxiety is often voiced during conversation with the nurse, rather than being withheld until the chaplain is present. Such patient demands for spiritual meaning may be sprung on the nurse at the most unlikely times and in the most unusual places. As mentioned earlier, not every nurse has a capacity to help patients meet specific spiritual needs.

Many a nurse rightly feels that she cannot reinforce a patient's faith when she herself does not share his beliefs and values. For example, how can a nurse who is a non-believer sincerely reassure a dying Christian patient of the presence of God? There are no easy solutions to such questions. A nurse without religious belief cannot reinforce a believer's faith. She can, however, help her patient to come to terms with his illness in an indirect way; by taking time to talk to him, being truthful, or listening to his worries, and trying to take positive actions to alleviate them.

Talking to the patient

Effective communication is a necessary prerequisite to the formation of any personal relationship. Without communicating with someone, it is impossible to know him as a person, touch his spirit, and be aware of his innermost worries. The reasons behind ineffective communication in acute nursing care situations are many and varied. Staff shortages and pressure of workload are undoubtedly contributory factors in busy surgical wards. The barriers to communication between a nurse and a patient of different nationalities, cultures and language are self-evident. Intensive care units pose a unique set of problems. No one undertakes communication with an unresponsive or unconscious patient with ease. Professional as well as lay people find it difficult to carry on a one-sided conversation with someone who is curarized, and mechanically ventilated. It is hard to remember sometimes that a spirit contained in a human being lies behind the seemingly moribund exterior. More difficult still is the situation where a person whose bodily life is being maintained by positive pressure ventilation, while his brain is officially and legally described as dead. Can we assume that the spirit has already departed from the body, or should the body be treated as though the spirit remained within it? All we can do is accept, with humility, that we will never know the answer, certainly not in this life, to such questions. A spiritual input, when applicable, must be included in the care, and the patient with brain death should be treated with the same degree of respect which would be accorded to any other human being. Anyone who comes to remove organs for transplant must be made to respect the body of the donor patient, whom they may not have known. The care of the spirit of the patient does not end abruptly at the moment of his death.

Truthfulness

It is difficult to imagine any aspect of nursing where truth is more important than in the area of spiritual care. Yet half-truths, or even lies, are often commonplace in respect of patients with a poor prognosis. Phrases such as 'Of course you're going to get better', or 'Don't be worried, you'll be home in no time', come from professionals and relatives alike. Why? Possibly because doctors rather than nurses decide how much information to impart to the patient concerning his condition, and the honesty of the nurse, therefore, is held in constraint. Another possible reason is that a much deeper level of conversation is demanded from the nurse if the patient faces the prospect of dying in truth. Many nurses are afraid of such a level of involvement, which often includes candid talk about death and the hereafter. The only honest way that any nurse can answer such searching questions, such as 'Why me?', is to humbly admit that she does not know the reason why. After all, God is the Creator, and we are all His creatures. Is it therefore really surprising that we fail to understand the workings of His purpose regarding suffering? Where a Christian nurse and patient share a bond of mutual faith, such problems can be dealt with in the light of Christian values, and the nurse is in a position to assure her patient of the love and steadfastness of God.

A personal view held by the author is that the truth should be spoken at all times. Lies, when uncovered, can do much to undermine a patient's confidence in the person responsible. Worse still, how can anyone come to an acceptance of a situation if he is denied the opportunity to face it truthfully? A patient in such a state may find that he must find peace with God against a tide of opposition from well-meaning persons. There is, of course, a place for sympathy and reassurance, but only if the truth of the situation is faced and the patient is not pressurized by being forced to live in falsehood.

Active listening

The importance of being a good listener cannot be overemphasized in respect of spiritual care. The active listener attends carefully to what the patient says and to what he does not say, detecting any note of depression, such as a sigh of resignation, or tears of despair. Often, advice to the patient is unnecessary, and the patient just needs a responsive listener whilst he sorts things out in his own mind. In cases of people facing death, Kubler-Ross (1969) claimed that a healthy acceptance is achieved when patients, 'have been encouraged to express their rage, cry and express their fantasies ... to someone who can sit quietly and listen'. Mere companionship from a caring person is reassuring in itself. There is no substitute for loving concern and, in whatever situation, it is important to avoid the temptation of giving inappropriate advice.

Summary

This chapter has examined briefly the declining emphasis placed on spiritual care in acute illness. A number of problems have been identified, including an acknowledgement that nurses vary greatly in their capacity to meet personal spiritual needs. As a limited solution, different levels of care have been suggested, ranging from basic facilitation of religious practice to the special personal ministry which is possible when a nurse and patient share a mutual faith.

The spirit of man is intangible by nature, even though its actions can be observed by outward phenomena. It must be said in conclusion, therefore, that although certain spiritual needs in a patient may be ascertained, the actual results of spiritual care given are very difficult to determine. The hospitalized patient will normally show evident signs of progress or deterioration. A patient who has been acutely ill may, however, begin to experience joy, peace or inner security long after his hospitalization.

A second, and related point is that the giving of spiritual care requires a good deal of motivation on the part of the nurse. Spiritual care will always remain a 'grey area' without either scientifically applied methods, or easily observable results. The individual spiritual beliefs and convictions of the nurse are, therefore, of major importance both in undertaking spiritual care, and in sustaining it with perhaps no visible reward at the end.

References

Autton, N (1980) The role of the hospital chaplain, Nursing Journal, 16: 697

Hall, C (1982) Approaches to Nursing Practice, Proceedings of International Intensive Care Conference, Macmillan Journals

Kubler-Ross, E (1969) On Death and Dying, Macmillan

Lewis, C S (1971) The Four Loves, Fontana

Lewis, C S (1982) Mere Christianity, Fontana

Lewis, L (1976) Planning Patient Care, 2nd Edition, William Brown

Further reading

Berger, P (1969)The Social Reality of Religion, Faber & Faber

Brand, P W (1974) Is Life Really Sacred? Christian Medical Fellowship

Myco, F (1983) Nursing Management of the Hemiplegic Stroke Patient, Harper and Row

Schaeffer, E (1979) Affliction, Hodder and Stoughton

Tournier, P (1957) The Meaning of Persons, SCM Press

CHAPTER 11

SPIRITUAL CARE IN CHRONIC ILLNESS

Introduction

Caring for individuals suffering from chronic illness requires a particular perspective. For example, the care giver has to consider the temporal effect of the illness on the individual's social identity, and he or she must also accept the fact that a cure is unlikely, and that the person suffering from chronic illness must come to terms with an altered self-image imposed upon him, say a broken body, or altered social roles and relationships. The needs of the person suffering from chronic illness must therefore be seen from a perspective which includes the effect of the illness on the person's functional ability — physical, mental, and social — and from the point of view of the effect of the illness upon the individual's philosophy of life.

Every illness or crisis compels the person to turn in upon himself and consider his life (Tournier 1974). Because of this, the care giver cannot ignore the effect the illness will have on the person's own value system. A value system is that set of beliefs and hopes which motivate and direct a person through life. The system may be based on a belief in God, and on the person's relationship with God, or it may be based on the person's own strength of character, which provides him with confidence and the ability to direct and give meaning to his life. As each person's experience of life is unique, so the development of his particular value system will be quite distinct. In crisis situations when a person is required to find new strengths, the care giver must be prepared to help the person understand the meaning of his altered state in terms of this person's own philosophical perspective. In doing so, the person is able to enrich and strengthen his value system, thus equipping him to cope with other situations in the future.

The aim of this chapter is to explore what it means for the nurse to provide spiritual care to persons suffering from chronic illness. Such responsibility is based on the belief that the nurse's primary function is to ensure the individual and personal integrity of persons under her care. This embraces both meeting patient's physiological needs and supporting them in emotional, cognitive and spiritual areas of life. The nurse, therefore, cannot ignore the spiritual dimensions of a person's experience during illness if she is attempting to meet the needs of the person as an individual. Consideration will be given to the nature of spiritual care and how it might be defined from a nursing care perspective; the main feature of chronic illness will then be discussed; the final area to be covered will deal with the nurse's activity in the spiritual care of such patients.

Spiritual care

By accepting the need for spiritual care, one must begin with the premise that man is a creature with a spiritual dimension, his spiritual needs being viewed in relation with other, physical, psychological and social needs (Maslow 1970; Henderson 1966; Roper et al. 1980). If people are to be viewed as whole, then their moral, ethical, spiritual and religious values cannot be ignored by health workers. 'Spiritual', however, does not necessarily mean 'religious'. The difference between the two terms is described by Vaillot (1970), who interprets spiritual as comprising that essential principle influencing each individual, including the psychological dimensions of the person, whilst religion is seen more in terms of the ritual.

The primary aim of spiritual care, according to Henderson and Nite (1978), is to help the person attain peace of mind. This is seen as the objective of all health carers, and in some ways there can be no real distinction between what doctors, nurses, social workers and others do to help patients attain or maintain their peace of mind. Health workers are in a position to establish relationships with patients which encourage them to express the fears, hopes, and conflicts which have resulted from their illness state. They are also in a position to evaluate the extent to which the illness situation has shaken the individual's faith or value system, his hopes and aspirations, his ideas about the existence of God, life and death.

In order to help the patient attain or maintain peace of mind, the health worker must be aware that often sickness, or prolonged disability, symbolize a direct assault on the person's value system (Henderson and Nite 1978). As the person matures his values change. When illness strikes, the person's value system may be shaken and found to be inappropriate to support him in his particular crisis. It may be that the person's concept of God or his understanding of the spiritual dimensions of his life are stunted; that religious ceremonies are neither meaningful nor supportive, nor a source of strength to him. Health carers must be aware that a sick person may be experiencing such conflicts. This requires sensitive and perceptive handling, in order to help the person to express his fears, hopes and conflicts, as they are affected by his altered physical and psychological state.

The nurse's contribution in identifying spiritual needs

The nurse's contribution to the spiritual care of patients is made special by three factors. These are related to the amount of time she spends with the patient, the level of interpersonal contact at which she operates and her ability to identify the patient's spiritual needs.

Nursing staff have the opportunity to build up more meaningful relationships with patients by virtue of the fact they provide a round-the-clock service. Nursing contact time with patients is, therefore, potentially greater than that of any other health worker. This gives her more opportunity to observe for signs of distress in her patients, or a desire on their part to talk. She must also be available to listen to patients and to share in elements of his anguish and distress.

Because of the time they spend with patients, nurses also tend to be involved more with patient's daily experiences. In a study by Beland and Passos (1975) of the distance between people in interaction in the hospital setting, nurses were found to spend more time than any other worker in the 'intimate zone', that is a distance of up to 0.5 m (1.5 ft). This level of intimacy was seen as appropriate by patients, serving not only to meet their physical needs, but also to permit the more personal communication of deeper needs and fears. In this respect, the position of the nurse is seen as extremely important in ensuring that the patient is encouraged to express his spiritual needs if he so desires.

In addition to time and interpersonal contact, factors such as the nurse's education and experience, both in terms of her personal and professional experiences, may affect her ability to identify the spiritual needs of her patients. Most pertinent is the nurse's own level of spiritual awareness or receptiveness to the type of problems being experienced by the patient. Henderson and Nite (1978) feel that the more spirituality nurses have, the more comfortable they are in discussing spiritual questions and the more likely it is that others will confide in them. Some nurses are more spiritually aware than others, and it may be a personal quality of theirs to be able to encourage patients to talk about spiritual matters. However, a number of practical steps have been identified by Fish and Shelley (1978) and Henderson and Nite (1978) which nurses may follow and which help to equip them to deal with patient's spiritual needs.

From an interpersonal perspective, the nurse must first of all identify her own values, spiritual needs and religious beliefs. She must also know something of the main religions and the significance of religious ceremonies and practices. The extent to which the illness has affected the patient's spiritual awareness may be assessed by listening to the patient and his family as they talk about the illness situation, whether they express anxiety, fear or worry. The nurse should also be aware of any aspects of treatment which may run counter to the values of her patient, and must learn to accept attitudes and statements non-judgementally.

Practical considerations relate to the carrying out of religious rituals or ceremonies. A patient's peace of mind may be helped by performing such religious ceremonies as praying quietly, having communion, or Bible reading. This may involve providing patients with a quiet room in which to meditate, or pray, or by offering to read a portion of scripture to a patient. The nurse should also be aware of the religious significance of certain belongings of patients and treat such with respect; she must also respect the dietary habits of patients as another form of religious practice.

Features of chronic illness

The primary aim of spiritual care has been identified as helping the person suffering from sickness or disability to attain or maintain his peace of mind. However, for the person suffering from chronic illness or disability, a number of significant factors related to the nature of long-term illness affect the way in which spiritual care is provided.

Chronic illness has been defined by Strauss and Glaser (1975) as including all impairments or deviations from normal which have one or more of the following characteristics:

1 It is permanent.
2 It will leave residual disabilities.
3 It is caused by non-reversible pathological alterations.
4 It will require special training of the patient for rehabilitation.
5 It may be expected to require a long period of supervision, observation and care.

A feature of chronic illness clearly identified by Harris et al. (1971) was that most people suffering from chronic illness live in the community, supported by a network of family and friends. The primary aim of health services in this area ought therefore to be to provide one or more support services on a sustained basis to enable individuals whose functional capacities are chronically impaired to be maintained at their maximum levels of health and well-being (Brody 1977). The objective should be for the chronically ill to restructure their lives, taking account of their altered physical capacities. The nurse can play an important role in achieving this objective.

In an attempt to highlight the potential range of needs confronting the individual suffering from chronic illness and how these relate to his value system, two main areas can be developed: coping with an altered lifestyle, and grieving for the past.

Coping with an altered lifestyle

The most significant feature of any chronic illness is its effect upon the daily living patterns of the sufferer. Depending on the severity of the illness, the sufferer may be slightly incapacitated by his condition with the result that his lifestyle is but little altered. The person's value system, therefore, might be quite acceptable and appropriate to his expectations of life. On the other hand, another individual sufferer might have experienced the almost total collapse of his lifestyle, possibly caused by a severe coronary thrombosis, a cerebrovascular accident with resultant paralysis and aphasia, or a road accident leading to permanent disability. Such an attack on the person's physical integrity will have widespread effects upon his future functioning in society and on his personal value system.

Strauss and Glaser (1975) identify a number of features which were commonly experienced by people suffering from chronic illness. They noted that after the initial onset of the chronic condition time was spent in trying to prevent recurrences of the acute episode of chronic illness. This may necessitate changes in diet, work or leisure habits, and consequently may affect a number of people linked with the sufferer. Control of symptoms — such as pain, over-exertion or fatigue — and carrying out prescribed regimens also take over a significant portion of time. Often as a direct result of the curtailment of social habits and an increasing amount of time being taken up in health care activities, people find themselves socially isolated and lonely. The individual is also expected to cope with the insecurities of chronic illness, that is, not being able to plan holidays or engagements in the future, out of fear of an exacerbation of the condition.

How the person copes with his altered lifestyle may be influenced by the preparation and support he is given from health workers who are aware of the complexities of the situation. During the initial onset stage of chronic illness, that is the diagnostic or early treatment stage, the nurse must try to discover the extent to which chronic illness has assaulted the individual's value system, his conception of self, his aspirations and his hopes for the future.

Several authors have suggested that an important aspect of the patient's recovery is acceptance of his altered physical state. Tournier (1974) emphasized that acceptance of one's infirmity does not mean a passive acceptance and a giving in to disability; rather the more difficult task is that in realizing the altered limitations of one's body one does not allow that knowledge to cripple the spirit. If the person suffering from chronic disability begins to see his dependent body as a reflection of his dependent self then according to Tournier he cripples his spirit and shuts himself off from outside contacts, becoming hard and inadaptable.

A study undertaken by Kerr (1977) which looks at the process of adjustment to disability of a group of orthopaedic patients, also identifies the need for those suffering from physical dysfunction to learn how to set themselves new goals and new priorities. Such goals have to maintain the individual's personal integrity, societal value and be within the limitations of each person's altered physical capacities.

Werner-Boland (1980), herself a tetraplegic, vividly describes the problems confronting individuals who find themselves unable to hold a mental picture of their new physically altered, disabled self. She wrote that, 'Being disabled is like moving into a new house in a new neighbourhood.

Shortly after the move, one looks out expecting to see the same old familiar sights. It takes time before one can look out with the realization that there is a whole new world out there'.

Kerr (1977) identified five stages in the process of adjustment, commencing with the shock stage where the person's self-image is still normal, and where he cannot accept the fact that he will not recover normality. The person continues to expect to recover totally in the second stage, but begins to accept the reality of his altered physical condition, if only within the framework of believing that it is a temporary problem. The slow realization that the body has altered irreparably often brings the person to a state of acute anxiety and depression, where he mourns the loss of his former self. In order to overcome this third stage, the grieving stage, the person must begin to restructure his altered self-image in a way which is acceptable to him. An important prerequisite to the adjustment stage is the ability of the disabled person to remaster social skills and regain a sense of social competence in dealing with the real world.

Grieving for the past

Consideration of the effect of grief on the person suffering from chronic illness or disability is an important concept in relation to the identification of patient's spiritual needs. Werner-Boland (1980) has looked at the grieving response and feels that it is a common problem faced both by persons suffering from chronic illness and by the family. The chronic grief response of the ill or disabled, however, is described as quite unlike that which occurs when the loss is an object outside of oneself. There is no immediate end to the situation that produces the grief — there is no foreseeable closure or resolution. What is distressing for the person suffering from chronic illness is the fact that he is there to mourn his own loss. While mourning the loss of another can be alleviated by the routine of living taking over, the disabled person cannot get back to his own normality, neither can his family or close friends. Thus, not only does the newly disabled person have his own burden of grief, but he also feels the impact of others grieving for him and because of him.

Old age may also be a time of grieving, particularly in situations where it is accompanied by chronic illness or disability. Old age is commonly viewed as a time when the person reassesses his life whilst coming to terms with declining bodily functions and the realization that death is not too distant.

Jung (1971) preferred to view old age in a more positive way, contending that the last half of life has purpose of its own, quite apart from species survival, namely the development of self-awareness through reflective activity. Erikson (1963) also sees man's last developmental stage in terms of a summary of life, when the individual looks back with a sense of achievement or integrity, or alternatively with despair and a certain amount of remorse. Peck (1968) takes Erikson's system one step further, and argues that to achieve integrity in old age the individual must be able to develop the ability to redefine self, to let go of his occupational identity, to rise above bodily discomforts and to establish personal meaning that goes beyond self-centredness.

Care givers of the elderly disabled should therefore recognize the fact that some may be disappointed and disillusioned with their lives, their value systems may not have developed to cope with the problems of old age, or their spiritual integrity may have suffered a series of blows. Alternatively, certain elderly persons — although being disabled — may show signs of tremendous moral and spiritual strength and personal integrity. Such individuals can be a source of spiritual strength to health carers, encouraging them to be optimistic about old age and disability. Important competencies required by health carers working with the elderly disabled include an awareness of previous coping patterns and value systems of elderly patients; an understanding and appreciation of the time it takes to work through the grieving over lost abilities, and to ensure that health carers have an understanding of their own feelings towards old age and disability.

Nursing action

The primary nursing goal is to help the patient regain optimal self-care and independence, thus enabling him to live as a whole person. In the case of individuals suffering from chronic illness, the nature of the relationship between nurse and patient is often intensified by the fact that the patient may require support over a protracted period, not only at the physical level but also psychologically, emotionally and spiritually. The nurse should be aware of her potential commitment to such needs and know how to protect herself from becoming over-involved with the physical and emotional pain of certain situations. Her relationship with the patient should be seen as a dynamic one, with an inherent flexibility which will enable her to anticipate and meet the variety of needs confronting her patient.

The nurse should also realize the effect she as an individual can have on the experiences and perceptions of the patient. Both Tournier (1974) and Werner-Boland (1980) state that patients with chronic illness expect the nurse to share in their suffering and that, if the nurse despairs of the patient, then she is in effect abandoning him. In order to prevent this occurring, nursing action can be divided into three separate yet related areas. These comprise the nurse as a comforter, as a counsellor, and as a challenger to the patient suffering from chronic illness.

The nurse as comforter

In order to be of comfort to the patient, the nurse must be able to identify and meet his basic physical needs. Ideally, patient's nursing needs are identified through a process of individualized care planning, followed by the carrying out of prescribed nursing action (Grant 1979). For patients hospitalized for prolonged periods the nurse must be aware of the tendency to stop noticing changes in the patient's condition. Thus, careful attention to details of personal hygiene and physical comfort is a primary feature within the framework of providing spiritual care. It offers an opportunity for the reticent, shy nurse to have a reason to give a little squeeze of the patient's hand, or place a comforting arm around bowed shoulders.

By becoming aware of the patient's fears, the nurse can work toward protecting the patient's dignity and personal integrity, first by recognizing his humanity and worth. Many patients in long-stay institutions learn to grieve silently for their loss, and to cry without tears. Losing control of one's bodily functions, for example, may become tolerable through sensitive support from nursing staff. Nurses should also be aware of the effect such feelings of helplessness can have on the individual's self-identity. Werner-Boland (1980) described the loss of control of bodily function as, 'worse than feeling nothing because feeling helpless is the ultimate in psychic pain'. A pretence that such a lack of control is normal, or that nothing is happening, can be as devastating to the integrity of the patient as a thoughtless, sarcastic remark.

An awareness of the possible feeling of loss, isolation and loneliness that the patient's suffering from chronic illness may experience can also enable the nurse to comfort and provide an atmosphere which helps to keep the personality intact. The problem of isolation is particularly relevant in respect of hospitalized elderly, who are infrequently visited by their families, and whose contact with the outside world is restricted. For patients who have reached the final stage of life, perhaps burdened with memories of lost opportunities or frustrated with life, depression and a feeling of rejection can ensue and overwhelm them. Nursing staff working in long-stay wards should encourage family support, and those patients who have few visitors can be 'adopted' by voluntary workers, or other staff members, so that they will feel wanted and of value once more. Enabling the elderly patient to make decisions for himself, however small, is essential to counteract the alienation which leads to isolation and withdrawal. For example, does the patient actually want sugar in his tea or coffee? This is just as important to his spiritual well-being as a religious ceremony, because it recognizes his individuality, and if he cannot be viewed as an individual human being how can he be seen as an individual belonging to God?

The nurse can also act as a comforter by ensuring that patients are able to worship according to their particular faith. This may involve group or personal devotions on a regular basis or such simple actions as changing a nursing routine so that the patient can spend a little more time by himself to read Scriptures, or to pray, rather than getting involved in a ward activity.

The nurse as counsellor

By being aware of the stages the patient may go through before he can accept his altered physical state, the nurse may be able to understand and therefore be more able to support the patient in times of stress. The nurse should be aware of the patient's value system prior to the illness, and of the support system surrounding each patient, as well as the effect the illness will have on his social role. Armed with this knowledge, she may be in a better position to listen to the patient when he becomes frustrated or angry, and feels he cannot cope.

Many chronically ill and disabled people are cared for in their own homes, often by a single relative, usually the spouse or unmarried daughter. Cognisance of the spiritual needs of the carer are an integral part of caring for the spiritual needs of the patient. Unrecognized distress in the relative will militate against the adaptation and growth of the patient. When the patient is elderly, and perhaps senile, attention may focus primarily on the relative. The community nurse who stops over for a cup of tea, and offers a sympathetic ear, or insistently pursues a little relief cover for the relative, will also be helping to maintain the spiritual care of the patient in such circumstances. Even a devoted child will find it difficult to continue to love an incontinent, senile, even dangerous and violent parent, as fatigue, disgust and feelings of being trapped begin to emerge. Incidents of disruptive or aggressive behaviour may be signals for the need of comfort and support. Instead of dismissing or ignoring such behaviour the nurse must consider the possibility that the disruption is really a cry for help. The nurse should be able to develop the skill of recognizing that the patient or relative needs to talk to someone, either herself, another member of the health care team, or the hospital chaplain.

The nurse as challenger

It is important for the nurse to have a sense of patience and hope in working with the chronic sick and disabled. According to Werner-Boland (1980), when the nurse despairs of the other person, then she has essentially abandoned him. The nurse has communicated by her lack of hope that she believes that the physical state of the person which appears unsalvageable, is a direct reflection of the patient's inner self, i.e. his spirit. She should be aware of the difficulties she will experience in trying to maintain attitudes of acceptance, patience and hope in the recovery of some patients, as it is much easier to slip into a disinterested frame of mind as a defence against one's own feelings of discouragement and despair.

In order to act as a challenger to the patient experiencing disruption in his daily living patterns, the nurse must be willing to become involved. She should work against becoming rigid and viewing the problems thrown up by illness as insurmountable. She must also see her relationship with the patient as complementary and positive, rather than her giving, and the patient receiving, all. Again, she must know her patient well enough to decide what his potential self-care capabilities are so that she and the patient together may set realistic goals. To do this successfully, she will need the support of senior colleagues, such as nurse teachers and administrators, who can often recognize the young nurse's struggle to maintain optimism in what might be a depressing situation even for many older and more experienced nurses.

The experience of loss, disability and chronic pain need not be viewed solely in negative terms. Tournier (1974) sees illness as a time when the person has to turn in upon himself and examine his life. This process may be therapeutic if the patient is supported and is encouraged to share some of his suffering and fears with others. Again, because of her frequent and intimate contact with patients, the nurse must be aware that often the patient will look to her for support. There is always a temptation for the nurse herself to join with the patient in his moment of despair, because she too can feel the hurt of a broken body and shattered future. Neither should she dismiss the patient's requests for help by not taking them seriously, but she must learn how to cope with emotionally stressful situations where patients need to be helped to continue to fight and to hope, not merely to wish that things will get better, rather she must share in a belief with the patient that he will be able to make sense of his situation and retain his personal identity.

For those patients in despair, the nurse may face a formidable task in knowing how and where to start rebuilding. Her strongest resource is her own perception of the patient; if she is able to respect and relate to the person behind the dependent body, then she may be able to help the patient rebuild his value system. Such spiritual restructuring requires a team effort, however, not the least of which is the patient's family and friends. Simply sitting quietly by the side of the patient may be a useful starting point. Unfortunately, the process of socializing nurses militates against the learning of such a skill without feeling embarrassment or a sense of not fulfilling other nurse's expectations. Offering to read to the patient may be an alternative introduction. Recognition of the need to respond to any attempt at verbal or non-verbal communication by the patient is important. Too commonly does one see an elderly hospitalized patient call out to a passing nurse, who tosses a reply such as, 'All right Amelia! In a minute!', and passes on without a pause, and without even establishing eye contact with the patient. 'Amelia' will probably become even more anxious that she has not been 'seen' by the nurses. A pause, and the establishing of eye contact while giving explanation, or when asking questions of patients, take up so little extra time, and yet may contribute so much to the interpersonal relationship between patient and nurse.

When recognition is lacking, elderly patients may attempt to establish identity in terms of innanimate objects, for example, becoming over-possessive of 'my flowers', 'my chair' or 'my newspaper', etc. To encourage such a patient to begin to share some of his belongings and himself with other patients, the nurse should first begin by encouraging the patient to share with her.

Summary

The nurse's responsibility in meeting the spiritual needs of patients suffering from chronic illness is seen to revolve round ensuring the personal dignity of the individual and striving to maintain the spirit intact even though the body may be broken. It is important that the nurse is aware of the effect a state of dependency or an altered lifestyle can have on the individual's value system, the framework of which has developed to give meaning to his life. In such situations the nurse not only tends to a dependent body but she is caring for a vulnerable spirit.

The nurse works as one of a team of care givers but her relationship is special by virtue of the fact that she spends more time and is in more intimate contact with patients. She therefore must be aware of the responsibilities this privilege confers upon her. Such intimate contact may lead to over-involvement with the pain and anxiety experienced by the patient. The nurse may either distance herself by refusing to respond to the person behind the body or she can act in such a way where she protects herself by approaching the patient's care in a positive and dynamic way. By perceiving her role as one of comforter, counsellor and challenger, the nurse can ensure both optimal physical care and meeting his deeper spiritual need.

References

Beland, I and Passos, J (1975) Clinical Nursing, Third Edition, Macmillan

Brody, E (1977) Long-Term Care of Older People, Human Science Press

Erikson, E H (1963) Childhood and Society, Second Edition, Norton & Co.

Fish, S and Shelley J A (1978) Spiritual Care: The Nurse's Role, InterVarsity Press

Grant, N (1979) Time to Care, Ron

Harris, A, Cox, E and Smith, C (1971) Handicapped and Impaired in Great Britain, HMSO

Henderson, V (1966) Basic Principles of Nursing Care, ICN

Henderson, V and Nite, G (1978) Principles and Practice of Nursing, Sixth Edition, Macmillan

Jung, C (1971) The stages of life, in J Campbell (Editor), The Portable Jung; translated by R F C Hull, Viking Press

Kerr, N (1977) Understanding the process of adjustment to disability, in J Shibbing (Editor), Social and Psychological Aspects of Disability, University Park Press

Maslow, A (1970) Motivation and Personality, Second Edition, Harper & Row

Peck, R (1968) Psychological developments in the second half of life, in B Neugarten (Editor), Middle Age and Ageing, University of Chicago Press

Roper, N, Logan, W and Tierney, A (1980) The Elements of Nursing, Churchill Livingstone

Strauss, A L and Glaser, B (1975) Chronic Illness and the Quality of Life, Appleton-Century-Crofts

Tournier, P (1974) A Doctor's Case Book in the Light of the Bible, SCM

Vaillot, Str M C (1970) The spiritual factors in nursing, Journal of Practical Nursing, 20: 30

Werner-Boland, (1980) Grief Responses to Long-Term Illness and Disability, Prentice Hall

CHAPTER 12

SPIRITUAL CARE IN MENTAL ILLNESS

Religion is relevant to the assessment and care of the mentally ill. Just as one
can be physically or emotionally ill, one can be spiritually ill.
Schnorr (1983)

Historical origins and modern perspectives

The healing of mental illness is historically embedded in Christian rituals
and practices, although in previous centuries it was called 'the curing of
souls' (McNeil 1951). Religious activity constituted the dominant form of
early psychiatry, whereby priests and witch doctors performed rituals,
prayers and magic to drive out the demons which they believed to be the
cause of mental illness. As late as the sixteenth century, the mentally ill were
subject to beatings, torture and similar punishments in the effort to drive
the 'devils' out of the body of the insane. Many mentally ill persons were put
to death.

Twentieth-century psychiatry led to conflict with religion, and Sigmund
Freud was prominent in developing suspicion between scientific psychiatry
and theology. In his books *Future of an Illusion* and *Civilization and its
Discontents*, Freud put forward the view that Christianity was false, not
because it was based on wishful thinking, but because he could see no
reason for believing in it (Freud 1934, 1939). Freud saw religion as an
interim social neurosis out of which man must grow as he becomes educated
to cope with, and be more closely in touch with, reality.

Carl Jung, a distinguished contemporary of Freud, developed an opposing view, in that it was the absence of religion which was the chief cause of adult psychological disorders. Jung pointed out the benefits of religion to mankind. Supporting this view, Flower (1927) suggested that a religious response to a situation may be one way of providing a possible means of bringing that situation under control. In a similar vein, Bartlett (1950) saw religion as a way of helping to make sense of the world, and of providing a basis for coherent action, especially when it is necessary to go beyond the immediately available evidence in taking such action. The implication of such views is that religion is somehow a means of dealing with the problems and frustrations of life, which often leads to the construction of an imaginary world to meet these frustrations.

Modern Christian healing movements appeal to the authority of the New Testament of the Bible. There are 72 examples of healing in the Gospels, and Favazza (1982) claimed that the healing of mental illness was a significant aspect of Christ's ministry. So much so that throughout history certain holy shrines were established across Europe — for example, the shrine of St Dymphna (the patron saint of the mentally ill) at Gheel in Belgium, or the more famous shrine at Lourdes, in France. However, from the 100 miracles which are recognized by the Roman Catholic church as having taken place at Lourdes, not one involves the curing of mental illness.

Today, fundamental Protestant movements and the Roman Catholic church have groups within them which accept supernaturalistic healing practices. Catholic healers work with and praise their Protestant colleagues, while some Protestant healers emphasize the healing power of the ritual of confession. Vecsey (1978), in the *New York Times*, reported that, in America, some 2000 Catholic and Episcopal churches hold spiritual healing services. Today, the 'demons' might be claimed to be alcoholism, drug dependence, gambling and similar obsessions, which result in the emotional disorders prevalent in modern society. Sanford (1976) argued that emotional illness is often the result of pathogenic memories which are surrounded by a defensive shell, deep in the unconscious. Such negative remembrances can be replaced with God-inspired reconstruction of those memories.

Linn and Linn (1978) — both members of the Society of Jesus, or Jesuits, and with practical experience as therapists at the Wohl Psychiatric Clinic, in St Louis, Missouri — follow the basic premise that neuroses and common fears can be healed by working through the four emotions of anxiety, fear, anger and guilt. They proposed the use of five stages of therapy, which are identical with the five stages of dying espoused by Kubler-Ross. Linn and

Linn also list with approval the 12 steps suggested by Alcoholics Anonymous for recovery from alcoholism, and point out that these steps parallel the steps necessary to recovery from the depression stage of anger.

Critics of religion still exist within psychiatry. Sullivan (1962) claimed that religion is, 'not so different from delusions', while Graves (1983) used these views to conclude that religion is a prominent base from whence spring delusional content. For example, Murphy and Vega (1982) found that first-time admissions for schizophrenia in Northern Ireland are significantly higher among Roman Catholics than for the rest of the population. For evidence of religious involvement in mental illness, critics also point to the large number of mentally disturbed, especially schizophrenics and depressives, who suffer from theopathic delusions. Religionists reply to such criticisms by reiterating that theoretically psychiatry lacks an adequate concept of the nature of tenderness. On the practical side, the psychiatrist finds himself unable to supply the love which his patients need, nor to receive the love that the patient wants to give. This is highlighted in transference during psychiatric treatment. Transference must be avoided, and broken when it occurs. By contrast, religion offers an interpretation of life, and a rule for life based wholly on love. Having rejected the religious approach to the cure of souls, science regards it as more realistic to centre attention upon the creative conditions of the mind — for example, hate, aggression and compulsive sexuality — even if these are merely the pathological conditions caused by deprivation of love.

Regardless of the divisions between religion and psychiatry, both groups coexist in the care of the mentally ill. Chaplains now study psychology, and in recent years psychologists have stressed the needs of the child for love in the home. Also, most religionists encourage persons with mental-health problems to seek psychiatric intervention. Conflict between psychiatry and religion is becoming less evident, and authors such as Jeeves (1976) believe that psychology and religion, when properly understood, are allies rather than enemies.

Spiritual needs in mental illness

Some of the more serious mental illnesses often manifest in the holding of bizarre ideas. For example, in acute schizophrenia and depression, expressions of attitudes, beliefs and religious rituals are commonly seen symptoms. Such themes include guilt, hopelessness, despair, unworthiness, self-depreciation, alienation from God, deserving of punishment, and inferiority. The following brief selection of cases illustrate recognizable manifestations in which spiritual needs are important.

Anxiety

Severe anxiety indicates the presence of some deeper problem, and apprehension, agitation and fear may overwhelm the patient. Comfort and peace are widely recognized as the fruits of spiritual care, and some psychiatrists acknowledge that simple religious observances can relieve tension and anxiety (Meares 1963). Uncondemning acceptance of the patient's fears coupled with assurances that he or she is not rejected are also aspects of the spiritual domain.

Suicidal tendency

Shame and a sense of rejection are common emotions found in recovering suicides. Pett (1973) claimed that such patients welcome the opportunity to talk with the chaplain of their choice. A friendly, uncondemning meeting is of inestimable value, even if the patient allows conversation to progress no further than an exchange of superficial pleasantries.

Depression

Religionists interpret depression as stifled anger against life, or fate, which has taken away something that was valued. When expressed this way, the existential or spiritual nature of depresssion can be understood. This is not meant to deny that depression is also a psychiatric problem which frequently requires medical intervention. In severe endogenous depression, delusions of unworthiness, guilt and sin may dominate.

Hostile behaviour

Some psychiatric patients may continuously express hostility, agitation, self-mutilation, or aggression. Even if doctors and nurses maintain their patience and control, most chaplains are also willing to attempt an understanding as to what the patient wishes to communicate through his or her disturbed behaviour.

Bizarre religious delusions and hallucinations

Acute schizophrenic states often manifest themselves in the expression of bizarre religious delusions and ideas. Stafford-Clark (1979) illustrated such symptoms in a case history concerning a 23-year-old graduate woman, who began to develop doubts about her religious position and to fear that she had sinned against the Holy Ghost, for which she and the Devil were jointly responsible to God. She claimed to have heard God's voice reprimanding the Devil for his part in the affair, and telling him that his last chance of being received back into heaven had gone. On admision to hospital, this girl said that she had the obligation of sacrificing herself to save the Devil. Stafford-Clark tells how she refused treatment, tried to pull out her hair and sat with her mouth pursed for much of the day.

In acute disturbances such as this, psychiatric treatment offers the best hope for early relief from torment, and for eventual recovery. However, religious language and spiritual reassurance can offer support to the mysterious forces that the patient feels and may help him to rationalize the catastrophic change occurring in his personality.

Religious mania

Some mentally ill patients are openly obsessed and preoccupied with religion to such an extent that they may dress in black clothing, decorate their bed tables with holy books, pictures or emblems. Some may wear rosaries or large crucifixes about their person and pray incessantly throughout the day and night. This condition may be chronic. Pett (1973) suggested that it would be kind and thoughtful to introduce overly religious patients to the chaplain as soon as possible after admission to the hospital.

Psychopathic behaviour

Irresponsibility, amorality, dishonesty, manipulation and pathological lying are features of patients with psychopathic or sociopathic disorder.

Inconsistency is another prominent characteristic. A psychopath may go to church in the morning, and by the evening he or she may be participating in theft or violent assault. He or she may help a blind person across the street on one occasion, but at another time may knock the same person down in the hurry to get somewhere.

According to Cleckley (1950) the psychopath is unable to experience shame, remorse or guilt. However, others have refuted this theory. At least, he appears not to learn from his past experience. Even though he may be punished and is intellectually able to distinguish between right and wrong, he does not seem able to carry out these concepts in real life. Spiritual care should avoid the temptation to moralize, or make judgement on the patient's behaviour regardless of how objectionable it may appear.

Possessive behaviour

In the long-term care of many chronically ill psychiatric patients, a Bible was one of the few personal possessions they were permitted to have in the past. The older, institutionalized patient, therefore, is usually very possessive of his or her Bible, and in some cases may carry it around so they can keep a watchful eye on it. The Bible is not only symbolic of the patient's religious views but serves as a useful container for precious photographs, letters, and other reminders of their earlier life. The Bible may offer the chronic patient one of the few opportunities to exercise autonomy, as he or she can govern, as well as maintain, full rights in its use.

Religion is a source of hope to many long-term patients, and guiding principles in group activities can have a religious base. These may include belonging to a caring community, finding security and sustenance in interpersonal relationships rather than attachment to a particular hospital ward, and experiencing a sense of group and personal history, with hope in future deliverance.

Spiritual care of the mentally ill

Schnorr (1983) claimed that nurses all too often limit the spiritual care of the mentally ill to asking questions about the patient's religious affiliation. Limiting spiritual care in this way ignores the wider purview of the spiritual dimension and may hinder the quality and effectiveness of care. Eddison

(1972) claimed that faith offers a vehicle others will seek. Patients do find relief through religious experience. The individual obtains a sense of identity, meaning and purpose from religion in addition to gaining strength, hope, support and fellowship. From this point of view, the nurse should be aware of the therapeutic potential of religion.

Religious counsellors can provide three elements in the counselling experience, which have been outlined by Crabb (1978) as encouragement, exhortation, and enlightenment. For the religious patient, their faith may be an important support system, and a significant resource in the recovery process. Adequate assessment and the planning of appropriate care intervention is essential to a holistic approach to the care of the mentally ill, but the nurse should be careful not to inflict his or her own moral code or value system on to the patient.

The assessment of the spiritual need of the patient should aim to establish the level and type of religious belief which the patient holds, and to identify ways in which the individual might benefit from intervention by nurses, religious advisers or chaplains. It is necessary to draw up a statement regarding the degree of devotion which the patient has toward a particular religious practice, especially if this could influence his behaviour or treatment. It is also important to establish whether the religious attitude is healthy. Rao and Katze (1979) outline guidelines for the assessment of healthy or sick religious attitudes and behaviour. These are as follows:

1 A sick religion acts as a vice: a healthy one reduces anxiety.
2 A sick religion deviates from the premorbid belief; a healthy religion is secure.
3 A sick religion differs significantly from others in the same belief system; a healthy religion is quite similar to others of the same faith.
4 An unhealthy religion may overwhelm the patient by false guilt; guilt determined by the opinions of self or others. The healthy religion defines guilt by the standards of God.
5 Like false guilt, false humility is seen in the sick religion. True humility is founded in self-acceptance, while false humility denies God-given personalities, abilities and resources.
6 A sick religion urges the denial of feelings, especially 'negative' ones. A healthy religion recognizes the universality of emotions and offers appropriate guides for their expression.

Should spiritual care of the psychiatric patient be left to chaplains? Piepgras (1968) argued not, and warned nurses not to dodge the spiritual component of care. Pumphrey (1977) stated that patients who enter hospital with their religious feelings can often have such feelings intensified by illness. It is now generally accepted that recovery and attitude toward treatment can be affected by the patient's religious beliefs.

In meeting spiritual needs, the nurse must also consider any emotional factors which are hidden by spiritual need or resources. The nurse should assist the patient to use the healthy dimensions of religion, support reality and help the patient in exploring and clarifying any points that may be considered as sick in his or her religious thinking. Nurses might be usefully guided by Stoll (1979) who claimed that nurses should consider four questions when they plan spiritual care; namely, what is the patient's concept of God? What is the patient's source of strength? What is the significance of the patient's religious practice? And what does the patient perceive as the relationship between spirituality and health?

Finally, chaplains satisfy a very definite need in the mentally ill, and it should be natural for the nurse to call for assistance. Although chaplains are usually willing to help in any way, whether or not a relationship will develop will depend largely on the initiative of the patient. The chaplain does not try to intervene, or to treat the patient in the medical sense, but by his presence invites the creation of a trusting and therapeutic relationship. The nurse should leave judgement as to the value or otherwise of such a relationship to those involved.

References

Bartlett, F C (1950) Religion as an Experience, Belief, Action, Oxford University Press

Cleckley, H (1950) The Mask of Sanity, C V Mosby

Crabb, J L (1978) Moving the couch into the church, Christianity Today, Sept: 1389–1391

Eddison, J (1972) The Troubled Mind, Concordia Publishing House

Favazza, A R (1982) Modern Christian healing of mental illness, American Journal of Psychiatry, 139: 6

Flower, J C (1927) An Approach to the Psychology of Religion, Kegan Paul

Freud, S (1934) The Future of an Illusion, Hogarth Press

Freud, S (1939) Civilization and its Discontents, Hogarth Press

Graves, C C (1983) Cause or cure, Perspectives in Psychiatric Care, 21: 27–37

Jeeves, M A (1976) Psychology and Christianity, Intervarsity Press

Linn, D and Linn M (1978) Healing Life Hurts, Paulist Press

McNeil, J T (1951) The History of the Cure of Souls, Harper & Row

Meares, A (1963) The Management of the Anxious Patient, Saunders

Murphy, H B and Vega, G (1982) Schizophrenia and religious affiliation in Northern Ireland, Psychological Medicine, 12: 595–605

Pett, Rev. D (1973) The hospital chaplain, Nursing Times, 20: 22

Piepgras, R (1968) The other dimension; spiritual help, American Journal of Nursing, 68: 2610–2613

Pumphrey, Rev. J B (1977) Recognising your patients spiritual needs, Nursing, 77: 64–70

Rao, A J and Katze, A (1979) The role of religious belief in depressed patients' illness, Psychiatric Opinion, 16: 39–42

Sanford, A (1976) The Healing Light, Trumpet Books

Schnorr, M S (1983) Religion: perspectives in psychiatric care, Point, 21: 1

Stafford-Clark, A C (1979) Psychiatry for Students, Allen & Unwin

Stoll, R G (1979) Guidelines for spiritual assessment, American Journal of Nursing, 79: 1574–1577

Sullivan, H S (1962) Schizophrenia as a Human Process, W Morton

Vecsey, G (1978) Spiritual healing gaining ground with Catholics and Episcopalians, New York Times, June 18

CHAPTER 13

SPIRITUAL CARE IN MENTAL HANDICAP

Introduction

When a mentally handicapped child is born, a crisis arises within the family group, and experience shows that, all too often, insufficient support is given to the parents in relation to the problems and difficulties which they will encounter. To give a medical diagnosis and then leave the parents to effect their own destiny at such a time is unwarranted. Yet health care professionals can, and do, allow this kind of thing to happen. This can be attributed, perhaps, to the fact that the advisers, or professionals, are unsure or even ignorant of what is the right thing to do. The parents require time to think, time to discuss, time to disbelieve, and then time to begin to believe. They may need the loving care and understanding of their faith and church, represented perhaps by a minister of a particular religion. Health care professionals should not shun any support at such a time.

Parents may feel cheated, and sometimes consider that God is paying them back for some wrong they have done. There is often a deep sense of guilt on the part of parents, and they may not always be able to confide this to a professional person. Consequently, the parents should be encouraged to talk to someone in whom they have a deep confidence, especially when they need to have their questions answered truthfully, and keep their hopes high within the bounds of probability. The church person does not need to assume the role of prophet, but rather that of a helper, and a source of understanding support for the parents, for months perhaps years to come.

In the modern world of caring for the mentally handicapped emphasis is placed on teamwork, but insufficient time and thought is sometimes spared to ensure that all team members are given opportunity to play their part. The part which might be played by the clergyman is sometimes overlooked; but my own experience has been that churchmen are always willing to be of help, but they are not asked or not made aware of the need often enough.

Attitudes of society to mental handicap

Before considering the provision of spiritual care for the mentally handicapped, it is necessary to establish a baseline from which to move forward. Such a baseline must inevitably include the past and present attitudes expressed towards this group of people. Such attitudes appear to arise from the fear and ignorance associated with lack of knowledge as the possible cause of the handicap.

The causes are many and varied, but can be divided into three main groups: those caused before birth, those caused at birth, and those resulting from incidents after birth. Children may be born already suffering from mental handicap because of genetic or chromosomal disorders. At birth, the handicap may be caused by injury — for example, forceps delivery, breech delivery, or cerebral anoxia. After birth, childhood diseases such as measles can lead to complications such as meningitis or encephalitis, which if unsuccessfuly treated can give rise to brain damage and mental retardation.

History shows that society has not always been as tolerant of the mentally handicapped person as it is today, in some parts of the world. Lack of insight continued until the early twentieth century, imbibed in the use of terms such as idiot, imbecile, moron and feeble minded as official categories for the mentally handicapped. As society became more knowledgeable, such offensive terms gave way to classification according to intelligence quotient (I Q) — for example, high grade, medium grade and low grade. Again, not generous terms but a considerable improvement on those previously used. During recent decades, the categorization, although still linked with IQ, has become even more explicit. The World Health Organization's current recommendations are as follows:

Category	Intelligence quotient (IQ)
Borderline mentally handicapped	52–67
Moderately mentally handicapped	35–51
Severely mentally handicapped	20–35
Profoundly mentally handicapped	below 20

Mental handicap, retardation, deficiency and subnormality are terms used in different parts of the world to describe the same categories of afflicted persons. Until recently, the term 'special care' (meaning people in need of special care) was used in Northern Ireland. Although a term which could be highly recommended, it was dropped because it caused confusion with the term 'Special Care Baby Units'.

If such was the official attitude to the mentally handicapped, what is the attitude of the public at large? Attitudes of the general public have changed dramatically, and for the better, over the last 20 years; but there is still a long way to go and a great deal more to do. A survey was carried out some years ago in France, Belgium, and French-speaking Canada to ascertain the attitudes of people in so-called normal society toward the mentally handicapped. The survey was carried out by three priests, one from each country, covering 85 parishes in all. Some of the findings are as follows:

1 Eighty eight per cent of the study population felt that all mentally handicapped people should be cared for in an institution, and should not be living in the community at all.
2 Sixty per cent considered them to be religious, and God's children.
3 Thirty per cent of the study population living in urban areas considered the mentally handicapped to be generous, compared with 20% in rural areas. Fifteen per cent, and 18% respectively, considered that they were selfish individuals.
4 Only 15% from urban communities would find mentally handicapped children living in their neighbourhood acceptable. Forty four per cent of those living in rural areas said they would be accepted, even welcomed in their neighbourhood.
5 Twenty four per cent of the priests interviewed in city areas considered the mentally handicapped to be honest and well behaved, but 27% considered that they had delinquent tendencies. In country areas, these percentages were 57% and 35% respectively.
6 Sixty per cent of priests considered the handicapped as being totally unable to take part in society, especially in rural areas. Only 21% of priests felt that they had a contribution to make. Among the adult mentally handicapped in this survey, 15–17% were found to have an interest in religion, and were religiously active, but nearly 44% were looked upon as being indifferent to religion.

In respect of the findings on the claimed tendency towards delinquency among the mentally handicapped, it must be pointed out that they are a vulnerable group of people, and easy prey for the unscrupulous members of society.

Clearly, there is still considerable insight required when it comes to discussing religion and the mentally handicapped. A number of questions have got to be asked. For example, what is the attitude of the local community to the mentally handicapped being involved in religion, and possibly attending their church? Is it at all possible to provide religious education for the mentally handicapped; and if so, who is to be responsible for providing it? Should it come from the family, clergy or school teachers?

Concerning the provision of religious education, it might be suggested that a combination of all three would be ideal; but given that children of different denominations attend schools for the mentally handicapped, it might bring about a situation whereby members of teaching staff could feel inadequate. Therefore, perhaps, the greater onus must be on ministers of religion, and parents, while not totally repudiating the teacher's role.

Assuming that a sizeable percentage of mentally handicapped persons, for example those at the upper end of the IQ scale, are able to appreciate and take advantage of religious practices, should they be taught in a formal setting? If the answer is yes, should teaching take place with their peer group, or with other children? If there is to be an attempt at normalization, then perhaps teaching should take place in a mixed-ability group. However, learners who suffer from mental handicap do tend to feel disadvantaged in the company of any average learner, and learning in the company of their own peers is possibly a more useful experience.

In order to find answers to such questions, and to try to overcome prejudice toward the mentally handicapped, special pastoral centres have been set up at regional level in several countries. Such centres have generated tremendous interest in their attempts to provide a religious dimension for the person suffering mental handicap. Countries which have taken great strides in this respect include Belgium, France, Canada, the USA, Britain, Ireland, Switzerland and Spain. In addition, in recent years, conferences on the subject of religion for the mentally handicapped have taken place in Rome, Vienna, Caracas and Montreal. Through such activity, much clearer recommendations have been made by the Christian churches — to people generally and to the Church hierarchies in particular — offering guidelines on such things as the receiving of sacraments, the age of sense and reason and the education of the mentally handicapped in religion. The right of the mentally handicapped to receive religious education is not questioned by churchmen, but, as yet, suitable levels of educations are not generally available. However, evidence of progress is noticeable in many of the Protestant faiths, who have established, or are in the process of establishing, specialists in the field of religious instruction and education. For example, the Lutheran Church in the USA has taken steps to offer a religious ministerial service to the mentally handicapped, through the adaptation of various tracts and with brochures and pamphlets which give a tremendous amount of information to those who wish to provide a religious service to the handicapped. A taskforce for special ministeries was set up by the National Council of Churches of Christ, also in USA, which proposed curricula materials for children, young people, and adults; much of which could be easily adapted to meet the needs of the handicapped. One current important organization in the USA is the National Apostolate for Mental Retardation. This body was established by the Roman Catholic Church and is an exemplary service promoting religious education amongst the mentally handicapped and their families.

Spiritual care in mental handicap

Questions are sometimes raised regarding the ability of the mentally handicapped to accept religion and to participate in church functions. Parents are justifiably worried and concernerd about the intellectual capacity and ability for learning in their children. But do the mentally handicapped have to be educated, and learn, before they develop an appreciation of their church and its religious services? It is extremely difficult to set criteria to the religious capacity of mentally handicapped people. If they are in any way receptive and willing to practise their faith, and the parents or guardian agree, then the professional person and the church hierarchy should attempt whatever is necessary to be accommodating. Too many pastors and parents have distorted views of their own faith as it applies to the mentally handicapped and tend to consider them on a similar plane to themselves. However, there are still many thousands of handicapped throughout the world who have been refused the right to religion, because they are seen not to be able to function on the same plane as others. In fact we should not even stop to consider their ability to reason, or to express their beliefs verbally. The Bible, for instance, does not give any event where Christ discriminated between the mentally handicapped and others. The mentally handicapped person's ability to enter into a relationship with another person should be sufficient evidence to allow him to enter into a relationship with his God. This should be acceptable, especially in the Christian churches, since Christians are taught to see Christ and the image of God in each other. Nevertheless, many people believe that religion is much too abstract a subject to be delivered to the mentally handicapped. This poses the question, is a supernatural thing necessarily abstract? Surely, faith, prayer and participation in one's church is not abstract. There are many ways to meet one's God, and as nurses we should encourage in every possible way a mentally handicapped person's search for God. When presented by the question, 'Who is God?', or 'Who is your God?', each human being, even the handicapped, will have a different perception of their God, and who is to say which is the correct one?

Reality must be faced, however, and it cannot be denied that if tradition is to continue and old catechetical methods retained, then many mentally handicapped persons are not educable in the field of religion, as most people know it. If religious education is a matter of learning, and not of living out one's religion by example taken from others, it has to be accepted that the person suffering mental handicap will be unable to learn to the level of the ordinary, but he can live in a loving relationship with his God, given the opportunity and the encouragement he requires within his capabilities. It would be folly to suggest that there is some magic means available to provide religion and faith in the field of mental handicap. We must consider them as persons first and foremost, and then proceed to provide religion as they are able to perceive it. If a mentally handicapped person's thinking is considered to be developmental, then so too must be his education and instruction in religion; and if, in time, effort and determination coupled with application are the hallmarks of success then the outcome will be positive.

The suggested developmental approach demands that the mentally handicapped person, whether child or adult, be given the chance to display and convey, by whatever means of communication is open to them, their own past experiences, needs and interests, and have these features utilized as the starting point for religious learning. It follows that a person's acquaintance with religious concepts should result from him being encouraged to look more deeply into his own feelings, actions and experiences, and to express what he discovers, in his own everyday language. Therefore, no opportunity should be missed to link the person's own experiences with whatever he discovers is his own central concept of religion, especially the implicit or feeling side of religion. The outcome should be not only a special way of looking at the talking about religion, but also a special way of talking about the experiences of life. The process of development is all embracing and includes social, emotional and physical dimensions, in addition to cognitive ones.

Mentally handicapped people will never be able to come to terms with the intelligent, intellectual aspects of formal religious concepts, but they are capable of having initiative and retaining knowledge despite the fact that they may not be able to convey this in an articulate manner. This points to the great importance of the implicit, or feeling side of religion; that is, experience becoming the core of religious experience. Given that the mentally handicapped do not have much choice about how and what they learn, those involved in the field of religious education need to accept that in the early stages the foundations must be laid on the person's social experience, with less concern placed on purely cognitive development.

In Northern Ireland, in 1975, Father John McCullagh established a group of catechists in Londonderry to examine the religious needs of the mentally handicapped. A number of pamphlets emerged from the group, including *Introducing the Mentally Retarded to the Eucharist* (McCullagh) and *The Religious Formation of the Mentally Retarded Person Within Selected Faith Communities* (Boyle).

The group established a project, starting with ten children, four girls and six boys aged between 9 and 17. Four of the children suffered from Down's syndrome and the others were brain damaged to varying degrees. Some were overactive and displayed aggressive tendencies, and their mental ages ranged from 2½ to 6 years. Through working with these children and learning from their reactions a large number of mentally handicapped people, who might have missed the opportunity, have now received the Sacrament of the Eucharist, and have learned to appreciate its significance within their religion.

A considerable amount of groundwork was necessary to test the capabilities of the children in the project, and this involved the parents, not all of whom were enthusiastic. In fact, family opinions were often divided on the issue of whether the mentally handicapped should be presented to receive the Sacrament. However, eventually people began to realize that it was a worthwhile exercise, and that a human right was being met when the handicapped received instruction in the faith of their family.

It is not surprising that the parents should need so much encouragement, for it is only when all those involved in the care of the mentally handicapped, including nurses, broaden their own perspectives, that a way to better understanding and cooperation will be open. All parties will need to display more harmony and greater flexibility in their daily management of the mentally handicapped. From my own experiences in caring for these special people, I feel that in many ways the subject of religion has gone into hiding. This is unfortunate, because it has such a steadying influence, and has such an air of tranquility about it, that its application and adaptation to the mentally handicapped can only be for the good of all involved, including those involved directly in their everyday care. I do not think that anyone would disagree with the Jay Report (1979) when it states that, 'We believe that all mentally handicapped people have the right to be treated as individuals, to live life to the full and to have access to the same services as normal people'. If we accept this statement, then we must not overlook the importance of spiritual care. In this connection, I recall a parent saying, 'There is light where before it was dull and grey and all is due to just that little bit of help'. Many opportunities for contact and cooperation between parents and professionals are not always grasped. All parties are usually well meaning in their actions, but intention alone is not always enough. More effort should be made in a practical sense to help each other to help the handicapped.

Those who wonder about the importance of religion in the life of the mentally handicapped might be helped by this little prayer:

Blessed are you who take time to listen to difficult speech,
For you help us to know that if we persevere we can be understood.
Blessed are you who walk with us in public places and ignore the stares of strangers,
For in your companionship we find havens of relaxation.
Blessed are you who never ask us to 'hurry up',
And more blessed are you who do not snatch our tasks from our hands to do them for us,
For often we need time rather than help.
Blessed are you who stand beside us as we enter new and untried ventures,
For our failures will be outweighed by the time when we surprise ourselves and you.
Blessed are you who ask our help,
For our greatest need is to be needed.
Blessed are you who help us with graciousness, who do not bruise the reed and quench the flax,
For often we need the help we cannot ask for.
Blessed are you when by all these things you assure us that the thing that makes us individuals is not our peculiar inner selves, not in our wounded nervous systems, not in our difficulties in learning,
But in the God-given self which no infirmary can confine.

Be glad and rejoice to know that you give us an assurance that could never be spoken in words,
For you deal with us as Christ dealt with all his children.

This prayer could only be described as a tribute paid by the mentally handicapped to all with whom they come into contact in their everyday living. Each of us must ask ourselves whether we are deserving of such a tribute.

There is obviously a great readiness on the part of the mentally handicapped to receive the normal of society into their lives. By the same token we should, perhaps, be more ready to receive them into ours. Services for the handicapped have greatly improved in recent years, but the area of religion in their care is one aspect which has tended to be overlooked. Spiritual care should be given a proper place in their everyday living, by the giving of more thought to providing a greater variety of choice for the handicapped. These people — wounded in body, mind and spirit — require the love, help and support that is typical of all religions throughout the world.

References

Boyle, D (1975) The Religious Formation of the Mentally Retarded Person within Selected Faith Communities, Diocesan Catechetics Commission, Pastoral Centre, Derry, Northern Ireland

Department of Health and Social Security (1979) Report of the Committee of Enquiry into Mental Handicap Nursing and Care, Chairman: Peggy Jay, Cmnd 7468, HMSO

McGullagh, J J (1975) Introducing the Mentally Retarded to the Eucharist, Diocesan Catechetics Commission, Pastoral Centre, Derry, Northern Ireland.

EPILOGUE

In the foregoing discussion we have attempted to reveal the importance of the relationship between religion and patient care. We have attempted to show that religion, although concerned with something beyond the observable events of everyday existence, is important and not peripheral to the everyday business of human activity. We have seen that religious teaching helps man to answer basic questions about life, and death, and the unexplained happenings in the world around him. With many others, we have argued that acceptance of religious teaching helps man to accept situations in which the established practices, of the sociotechnological world, have been found wanting. We have seen that ill people, and their intimates, are especially susceptible to certain basic problems of human existence, which bring them face to face with situations in which established and extraordinary practices have been found wanting. In this connection, we have attempted most of all to stress the importance of attitudes belonging to what might be termed 'spiritual support' in any nurse–patient relationship.

Here it may be noted that we have no more than hinted at the occupational role of any nurse — in the sense of offering spiritual support to any patient. We have, rather, concentrated on features of religion itself, and its relation to certain features of illnesses, and the notion that the spiritual aspects of the patient can only be neglected at the risk of some damage to his integrity. Here then, by way of postscript, is a short discourse touching an area of possible difficulty facing any nurse within the concept 'Nursing and Spiritual Care'.

The area of possible difficulty centres around a point of tension between acceptance of matters of faith and those of knowledge for the well-being of any patient.

The Committee on Nursing (Department of Health and Social Security (1972), Chapter 1, para 13) states:

> We are in full agreement with the statement made to us ... by the General Nursing Council for England and Wales, first that, the role of the nurse must always be closely related to the needs of patients, and second that, these needs are never static, but vary according to individual patients; medical and technical advances and developments such as the possibility of a unified nursing service. Thus the role of the nurse is continually changing... .'

This may be interpreted to mean that the function of the nurse centres on her responsibility for caring for the patient in the sense of helping him in activities that are related to health. And in meeting this responsibility she is expected to acquire and use competence in the science of nursing and the techniques based upon it. In fact, it might be taken that nurses can depend on a set of principles common to any nurse–patient process, and that nursing practice is supported by a systematized set of rules designed to meet not only the obvious problems faced by the patient, but also a wide range of less obvious difficulties and potential complications open to any patient. Yet, regarding the integrity of any patient's needs, an important aspect of professional nursing is that each part of the nurse's task contains a discretionary feature. Discretion cuts across all the tasks carried out by the professional nurse; even those tasks carried out by the most junior nurse. In common-sense terms, however, it would appear possible to see nursing practice as a range of activities organized about the application of scientific knowledge by technically competent, trained personnel.

However, there is also the view and confidence of wider society that the professional nurse is ethically as well as technically competent. Also, according to tradition, her moral and spiritual values influence the way the nurse performs her duties and how she cares for the people in her charge. The International Code of Nursing Ethics, adopted by the International Council of Nurses, states:

> Nurses minister to the sick, assume responsibility for creating a physical, social and spiritual environment which will be conducive to recovery and stress the prevention of illness and promotion of health by teaching and example ... . The fundamental responsibility of the nurse is three-fold: to conserve life, to alleviate suffering and to promote health.

Seen in this broader perspective, the role of the nurse becomes significant not only within the bounds of the common-sense definition of the functions of the nurse in relation to health, but also includes relations to such things as the 'sacred rights of life' and the 'quality of life'. These are matters of vital interest to all people who are concerned about human well-being. Yet, in the practice of her profession, the nurse faces such matters in a very real way. Thus we find an area of possible difficulty facing the nurse within the concept 'Nursing and Spiritual Care'.

The nurse is placed at a point of tension between the supraempirical and the empirical; between acceptance of matters of faith and those of knowledge — most often in a knowledge-oriented place of work. She must work in relationship with both the sacred and profane points of view, and cope with both the ultimate and the ordinary. From this position the nurse, and the nursing profession, have always faced difficulty and have devised specific 'ways' of meeting the personal strains and overcoming the obstacles to effective nursing practice. Yet there is much more to be done!

Suffice it to say that increasing knowledge and technology, the tendency towards secularization and a readier acceptance of the views derived from it — together with greater decision-making within nursing itself — have probably created kinds of problems that would have been thought unlikely in the profession of a generation ago. Whether there are new kinds of problems to be solved, or a greater dilemma which cannot be eliminated but must be dealt with in some way, must concern present nurses. Since the significance of this area of possible difficulty — in both these respects — is still unknown to us, the outcomes of possible researches in this area are long overdue.

INDEX